The Heads-Up on Sport Concussion

Gary S. Solomon, PhD

Psychiatric Consultants, Nashville, Tennessee

Karen M. Johnston, MD, PhD

McGill University, Montreal, Quebec

Mark R. Lovell, PhD

University of Pittsburgh Medical Center, Pittsburgh, Pennsylvania

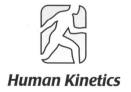

Human Kinetics

Library of Congress Cataloging-in-Publication Data

Solomon, Gary S., 1952-
The heads-up on sport concussion / Gary S. Solomon, Karen M. Johnston, Mark R. Lovell.
   p. ; cm.
   Includes bibliographical references.
   ISBN 0-7360-6008-1 (soft cover)
1. Brain--Concussion. 2. Sports injuries.
   [DNLM: 1. Brain Concussion--physiopathology. 2. Athletic Injuries--physiopathology. 3. Athletic Injuries--therapy. 4. Brain Concussion--therapy. WL 354 S689h 2006] I. Johnston, Karen M. II. Lovell, Mark R., 1953- III. Title.
   RC394.C7S65 2006
   617.4'81044--dc22   2005017701
ISBN: 0-7360-6008-1

The Web addresses cited in this text were current as of July 2005, unless otherwise noted.

Acquisitions Editor: Loarn D. Robertson, PhD; **Developmental Editor:** Anne Cole; **Assistant Editor:** Kim Thoren; **Copyeditor:** Amie Bell; **Proofreader:** John Wentworth; **Permission Manager:** Dalene Reeder; **Graphic Designer:** Bob Reuther; **Graphic Artist:** Angela K. Snyder; **Photo Manager:** Sarah Ritz; **Cover Designer:** Keith Blomberg; **Photographer (cover):** MTB©Christian Perret/Jump; **Art Manager:** Kelly Hendren; **Illustrators:** Andrew Tietz and Al Wilborn; **Printer:** United Graphics

Printed in the United States of America

10 9 8 7 6 5 4 3 2 1

Human Kinetics
Web site: www.HumanKinetics.com

United States: Human Kinetics
P.O. Box 5076
Champaign, IL 61825-5076
800-747-4457
e-mail: humank@hkusa.com

Canada: Human Kinetics
475 Devonshire Road Unit 100
Windsor, ON N8Y 2L5
800-465-7301 (in Canada only)
e-mail: orders@hkcanada.com

Europe: Human Kinetics
107 Bradford Road
Stanningley
Leeds LS28 6AT, United Kingdom
+44 (0) 113 255 5665
e-mail: hk@hkeurope.com

Australia: Human Kinetics
57A Price Avenue
Lower Mitcham, South Australia 5062
08 8277 1555
e-mail: liaw@hkaustralia.com

New Zealand: Human Kinetics
Division of Sports Distributors NZ Ltd.
P.O. Box 300 226 Albany
North Shore City
Auckland
0064 9 448 1207
e-mail: info@humankinetics.co.nz

"This book is a must-read for all coaches, parents, and yes, contact-sport athletes. Written by respected authorities and comprehensively and clearly covering the white-hot sports medicine topic of concussion, this book merits reading by all involved with sports."

Robert C. Cantu, MD, MA, FACS, FACSM
Chief of neurosurgery service and director of sports medicine,
Emerson Hospital, Concord, MA
Medical director, National Center for Catastrophic Sports
Injury Research

"This book provides a unique and much-needed perspective on the increasingly common problem of sport-related concussion. The book covers all aspects of sport-related concussion and will serve as an invaluable resource for physicians, athletic trainers, coaches, parents, and athletes. This book is a must-read for anyone interested in the issue of brain concussion in sports."

Joseph Maroon, MD
Team neurosurgeon, Pittsburgh Steelers
Heindle Scholar in Neuroscience
Professor, University of Pittsburgh School of Medicine

"This work by Solomon and colleagues provides for all of us an excellent shelf reference summarizing the current state of clinical practice and applied research related to the assessment and management of sport concussion. The authors have successfully created a valuable resource appropriate for all professionals charged with the care of athletes after a concussion. In contrast to other respected texts intended primarily for a medical readership, this introductory text also provides a wealth of information that athletes, parents, and coaches will find helpful as they attempt to gain a better understanding of concussion, the expected course of recovery, and the basis for a cautionary approach to return-to-play decision making after a head injury. The authors also offer a unique contribution to the literature with their dedicated section on injury treatment and rehabilitation, which is often lacking in the discussion on concussion management. By pointing out those questions yet to be answered regarding young sport participants' early and long-term risks, the authors admirably pave the way for future research that will continue to drive an evidenced-based approach to clinical management of sport concussion."

Michael McCrea, PhD, ABPP
Director, Neuroscience Center
Waukesha Memorial Hospital

"This book is a unique approach to understanding concussion in sport. The text is current and comprehensive in scope. All aspects of concussion, from anatomy and metabolism of the injury to assessment and treatment of injury, are discussed. As an athletic trainer involved in professional football, I was interested in the information about other professional sports. I found the writing style to be unlike that in a textbook; the information is presented in such a way that it was very readable and easily understood. In addition to being a valuable resource for the athletic trainer, the text will also be of value to parents who have children involved in sports as well as coaches and other health professionals."

John A. Norwig, ATC
Head athletic trainer
Pittsburgh Steelers Football Club

Contents

Preface vii

Acknowledgments xi

Chapter 1: Sport Concussion: Just the Facts **1**

Cast of Characters in Sport Concussion *1*
The Brain *4*
What Is a Concussion? *7*
Are Head Injuries in Sports Really a Problem? *12*
Second-Impact Syndrome *15*
Increased Awareness for Sport Concussion *17*
How Many Athletes Get Concussions? *20*
Research Digest *24*

Chapter 2: Brain Processes and Symptoms **25**

What Happens in the Brain During a Concussion? *25*
What Are the Typical Symptoms of Concussion? *31*
What Is the Role of Loss of Consciousness in Sport
     Concussion? *34*

Chapter 3: Assessment and Evaluation **37**

Clinical History *37*
Sideline-Assessment Strategies *38*
Balance Testing *42*
Neuroimaging Techniques *44*
Neuropsychological Testing *49*
Role of Grading Scales in Assessment *52*
How Long Does It Take to Recover
     From a Concussion? *56*
Research Digest *57*

Chapter 4: Treatment and Rehabilitation **61**

Medical Treatments for Concussion 61
Nonmedical Management and Rehabilitation 63
Research Digest 68

Chapter 5: Concussion in Professional Sports **69**

Concussion in the National Football League 69
Concussion in the National Hockey League 74
Concussion in Boxing 76
Concussion in Soccer 82
Research Digest 90

Chatper 6: Current Trends, Research, and the Future **93**

What Are Professional Organizations
      Doing About Sport Concussion? 93
What Are the Long-Term Effects of Concussion? 98
Do Helmets Help? 106
What Can We Do About Concussion? 109
New Research and the Future 110
Research Digest 112

Appendix A: Essential Information for Athletes,
Parents, and Coaches 115

Signs and Symptoms 117
Assessment, Evaluation, and Treatment...................... 118
Sport-Specific Concerns 120
Long-Term Effects 121
Return to Play.. 122
Educating Athletes About Concussion 122

Appendix B: Resources 125

References.. 127

About the Authors 139

Preface

This book began as a five-page "Introduction to Concussion" seminar presented to professional hockey coaches in 2001. We began to expand the information in an attempt to compile an introductory guide to concussion for athletes and their families, professionals, and patients who often have similar questions about concussion, treatments, and long-term outcomes. The material included in this book presents the final product after several years of compiling information on sport concussion.

Some excellent advanced medical textbooks are available on sport concussion (for example, see Lovell, Echemendia, Barth, and Collins, 2004, *Traumatic Brain Injury in Sports: An International Neuropsychological Perspective*). No introductory book on sport concussion, however, is directed specifically toward professionals who work with athletes. *The Heads-Up on Sport Concussion* is directed toward sports medicine and family physicians, athletic trainers, athletes, coaches, psychologists, students, and other professionals interested in sport concussion. Our hope is that the reader of this book will gain a more complete understanding of the various aspects of sport concussion and thus provide better care and education to athletes who sustain sport concussions. Although much of what is presented in this book may be applicable to concussion in general, the focus is on sport-related concussion. This book is not intended to be a substitute for appropriate medical or neuropsychological evaluation and treatment of any type of concussion. An athlete (and any other person) should always see a physician for the initial evaluation of a concussion.

The Heads-Up on Sport Concussion is a relatively comprehensive review of the current literature on sport concussion. The book includes information related to concussion and head injury from the fields of biochemistry, neuroimaging, neuropsychology, and epidemiology. We have made a conscious attempt to avoid dealing with detailed scientific critiques of the studies presented. We encourage you to consult the original sources if you would like more information about scientific methodology, data-analysis techniques, and experimental design. Most chapters include a Research Digest section to provide further scientific details of particular studies. Appendix A presents an overview of the content in chapters 1 through 6, with a special focus on the concerns that interest athletes, parents, and coaches. Clinicians can use this appendix as a communication tool when working with these individuals. Appendix B contains a resource section on sport concussion with a list of helpful Web sites.

Virtually all of the information contained in this book is based on the work of experts in the fields of sports medicine, neurology, neurosurgery, and neuropsychology. We have attempted to synthesize their scientific work into a readable and understandable introductory text. In an effort to make the text accessible for multiple levels of readers, we have included a running glossary that contains terms specific to the field.

We address the definitions of concussion, symptoms of concussion, short- and long-term effects of concussion, the demographic and epidemiological data on sport concussion (by gender and sport, when available), and what is thought to happen in the brain structurally and chemically during and after a concussion. We review grading scales, the use of neuropsychological and neuroimaging tests, and the role of loss of consciousness in sport concussion. We look at what the National Collegiate Athletic Association (NCAA), National Football League (NFL), and National Hockey League (NHL) have done and are doing about concussion. Overviews of concussion in boxing and in soccer are presented with a focus on heading the ball in soccer. Finally, various diagnostic and assessment strategies for concussion are addressed and consensus opinions about rehabilitation are presented. We have attempted to make it clear when we are presenting our personal opinions. We use the terms *concussion, closed head injury,* and *mild traumatic brain injury* (mTBI) interchangeably throughout the book, although in scientific parlance and clinical reality they are not necessarily the same.

Various chapters and sections in the book begin by posing a general question about an area of sport concussion. At the end of each section we offer conclusions and our opinions. We are also making a poster available for concussion education. This poster is a free download and can be found at www.HumanKinetics.com/TheHeadsUpOnSportConcussion. We hope that trainers, physicians, coaches, and sports medicine professionals will use this poster to educate athletes and their families about the signs, symptoms, and treatment of concussion.

The evaluation and treatment of sport concussion are rapidly expanding areas of sports medicine. New findings appear in the professional literature almost every month, so it is virtually impossible for the information in this book to be entirely up to date. However, every attempt has been made to keep the information in this book current and timely. With those caveats in mind, let's get to work.

Acknowledgments

We extend our appreciation to Loarn Robertson, senior acquisitions editor at Human Kinetics, for his willingness to publish our work and to Anne Cole, our editor at Human Kinetics, for making our manuscript readable and presentable.

For permission to use photographs and drawings we heartily thank Dr. David Hovda of UCLA; Dr. Richard Leblanc, Jen-Kai Chen, and Dr. Alain Ptito of the Montreal Neurological Institute; Russ Pace and Andy Solomon of The Citadel; Tom McClellan and Kip Sloan of East Carolina University; Laura Duncan of the Center for Research and Education at Centennial Medical Center; Matt Nelson, Teddie Whitaker, and Mark Cohen of Wofford College; Richard Riley; Brian Stutts; Nancy Solomon-Stutts; Cindy and Lionel Cartwright; Kristy and Katie Solomon; The Alzheimer's Disease Education and Referral Center; the National Institute of Health; and the National Institute on Aging. Appreciation is extended to Dr. Robert Jamieson for computer expertise and to Geoff Kaplan, ATC, of the Tennessee Titans for football terminology specifics.

To our families, friends, business partners, and office staffs who supported us through this endeavor, we offer our apologies and love.

We offer our respect and thanks to the athletes, coaches, athletic therapists, physiotherapists, trainers, physicians, and sports medicine professionals with whom we work in the area of sport concussion.

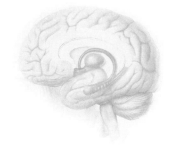

chapter 1

Sport Concussion: Just the Facts

In this chapter we discuss the people involved in the assessment and treatment of sport concussion; introduce you to some basic facts about the brain; and review some definitions of concussion, which is more difficult to pin down than you might think. We also discuss the demographics of sport concussion and review the available epidemiological data.

Cast of Characters in Sport Concussion

The cast of characters in sport concussion includes athletes, physicians, athletic trainers, sport psychologists, and neuropsychologists (now being called sport neuropsychologists by some authors). Let's get more specific about who these folks are and what they typically do.

The athletes discussed in this book include those involved in various high school, collegiate, and professional sports. We have little data to share regarding athletes younger than the midteens. In general, the information presented relates to athletes in the age range of 15 to 40. The studies reviewed include athletes of both genders, although female athletes have been studied specifically as a group in sport concussion only recently. Therefore, more data are related to men than women in the available literature. We predict this difference may disappear in the near future (particularly because women appear to incur more concussions than men do in some sports). See the chapter by Brooks (2004) for a discussion on gender issues in brain injury.

The care of athletes who have sustained a sport concussion is generally assigned to a team of sports medicine and health care professionals, which may include athletic trainers, physicians, and neuropsychologists. Responsibilities and duties among these professionals vary across settings and individual levels of training and expertise.

Physicians are major players in the assessment and treatment of sport concussion. Indeed, physicians typically have primary responsibility for medical care and return-to-play decisions. Team physicians at the professional level often include members of the medical specialties of internal medicine, orthopedic surgery, neurology, family practice, neurosurgery, ophthalmology, plastic surgery, and dentistry. Each National Hockey League (NHL) team seems to have a virtual mobile unit of physicians at each game, including an orthopedic surgeon, dentist, internist, plastic surgeon, and ophthalmologist. Most National Football League (NFL) teams have at least an internal medicine physician and an orthopedic surgeon on the sideline at each game. The suggestion has been put forward that a neurological specialist should be in attendance also. A primary care physician (PCP) is also a significant partner in this process, especially in the absence of a full-time team physician.

Although head injury and concussion have typically been viewed as being primarily within the scope of the medical specialties of neurology and neurosurgery in a hospital setting, it seems paradoxical that physicians of varying specialties have become involved in the evaluation and treatment of concussion in sports. It is possible that in many instances the physician's specialty may be less important than his or her knowledge about and experience with concussion.

The team athletic trainer (or ATC, which stands for athletic trainer, certified) is the front-line health care professional in sport concussion. Dr. Michael Ferrara and colleagues (2001) reported that ATCs care for an average of seven concussive injuries per year. It is the ATC to whom most athletes initially report their symptoms and concerns, and it is the ATC in whom athletes often have the greatest trust. ATCs who work closely with athletes generally know them best and are usually the source of an excellent opinion as to how an athlete is functioning after a concussion.

A neuropsychologist is a doctoral-level psychologist (PhD or PsyD) with specialty training and experience in the assessment and treatment of disordered brain–behavior relationships. A *neuro*psychologist (or sport *neuro*psychologist) is not the same as a sport psychologist. A sport psychologist is a doctoral-level psychologist who has specialty training and experience in the scientific application of psychological factors that are associated with participation and performance in sport and exercise. Kontos and colleagues (2004) have published an introduction to sport concussion for the sport psychology consultant. Neither a sport psychologist nor a neuropsychologist is a medical doctor, and neither can prescribe medication independently or admit a patient to a medical hospital.

Although both types of psychologists can make valuable contributions to athletes, their roles differ considerably. We recommend seeing a neuropsychologist for the evaluation and assessment of sport concussion and a sport psychologist for issues related to athletic performance. New data about the role of sport psychology interventions in concussion rehabilitation are being explored (Bloom et al. 2004). The neuropsychologist typically administers written, oral question-and-answer, or computer-based tests to evaluate the cognitive effects of concussion. In some settings, physicians and ATCs will administer cognitive tests; they should be properly trained and experienced in the administration and interpretation of these tests. Just because someone is licensed as a physician, athletic trainer, or psychologist does not automatically mean that the individual is competent in the administration and interpretation of cognitive tests used for the evaluation of sport concussion.

So this is the cast of characters in sport concussion. Who is the leader of this team of sports medicine professionals? Who makes the decision about returning an athlete to play after a concussion? In a survey of 339 athletic trainers attending the 1999 National Athletic Trainers' Association (NATA) Annual Meeting, Ferrara and colleagues (2001) reported that team physicians (40%) and athletic trainers (34%) were primarily responsible for making return-to-play decisions. Professionals have varying opinions as to who should take the lead and who should make the decision about an athlete's return to play after a concussion. Some maintain that the team physician should decide, whereas others think that the ATC should medicolegal—The interface of medical practice and legal (liability) issues.

make the call. Yet others believe that the neuropsychologist should make the decision. The politics and, more important, the **medicolegal** considerations surrounding this issue are significant. A simple, straightforward answer to these questions cannot always be found. The circumstances, resources, and professional expertise of the available sports medicine professionals of each team may dictate the answer. With all things being equal and under ideal circumstances, we believe that the final decision should be one of consensus among the professionals, as recommended by the NATA position statement on sport-related concussion (Guskiewicz et al. 2004). Ultimately, however, the final decision in most cases will be left to the team physician.

The Brain

The brain is the head coach, general manager, and chief executive officer of the mind and body. Like the human heart, it is always working. The brain, however, has a much longer life span than the typical career of a sports team head coach, general manager, or corporate CEO. The long life span of the brain is one reason to be concerned about an athlete's brain and to make every effort to protect it. The brain is the only one the athlete will ever have.

Concussion can impair the brain functions of thinking and reaction time (often referred to as speed of information processing), memory, concentration, balance, and eye–hand coordination. These abilities are the cognitive functions of the brain, and they are the most vulnerable in a concussion. A concussion can be as simple as a brief blow to the head, with rapid recovery, or it can be a life-threatening medical emergency. A concussion is an insult to the brain (both literally and figuratively). Figure 1.1 shows a side view of the major parts of the brain.

Athletes tend to show greater worry over an injury to a knee than to the brain. And yet, a knee can be repaired surgically; we cannot do this routinely with an injury to the brain. An athlete with a concussed brain can be a danger on the field, both to herself and to her teammates. Not all concussions are created equally, and all need to be considered individually. Both neurological and psychological factors are relevant and may need to be taken into

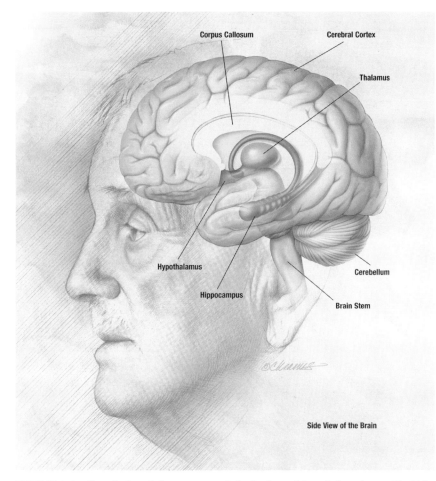

FIGURE 1.1 Knowledge of the structure of the brain and how it functions will aid in understanding concussions.

Courtesy of the Alzheimer's Disease Education and Referral Center, a service of the National Institute on Aging.

account in the assessment of concussion. The clinical evaluation of concussion requires an individualized approach, as recommended and described by the Concussion in Sport Group (2002).

Let's review some basic information about the brain. The consistency of the brain is similar to gelatin and thus is vulnerable to outside trauma. Figure 1.2 shows a lifelike model of an exposed human brain. It is encased within the skull, which offers it some protection. However, the skull does not absorb impact forces to the head, so it functions very poorly as a shock absorber. This lack of ability to absorb impact leaves the brain vulnerable to injury, and

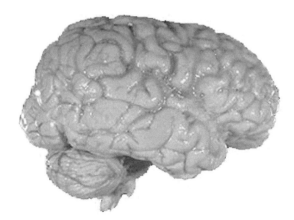

FIGURE 1.2   Model of the outside of the human brain.
Courtesy of the National Institute of Health. From http://www.nih.gov.

it is one reason why helmets and appropriate athletic technique are important.

The average weight of an *adult* human brain is about 3 pounds (about 1.4 kilograms). The average width is 5.6 inches (14 centimeters), average length is 6.68 inches (17 centimeters), and average height is 3.72 inches (9 centimeters). The brain constitutes about 2% of the total body weight. The brain is made up of two hemispheres, referred to as the right and left hemispheres.

The two hemispheres are near-mirror images of each other structurally, although they are quite different functionally. Each hemisphere is composed of four lobes, or sections, as illustrated in figure 1.3. The cerebellum, which is also depicted in figure 1.3, is the fifth area of the brain, but by tradition it has not been considered a "lobe" of the brain. The frontal lobes make up 41% of the total brain, and the temporal lobes account for about 22%. The parietal and occipital lobes account for 18% and 19% of the brain, respectively. The total surface area of the cerebral cortex (the gray, quarter-inch covering of the brain) is about 2.5 square feet (0.75 meters).

The composition of the brain is 77% water, 11% lipids, 8% protein, 1% carbohydrates, 1% inorganic salts, and 2% soluble organic substances. Because about three-fourths of the brain is water, you can appreciate why dehydration can be a life-threatening condition for athletes.

The average number of brain cells (nerve cells or neurons) is 100 billion. The average number of neurons in the cerebral cortex is

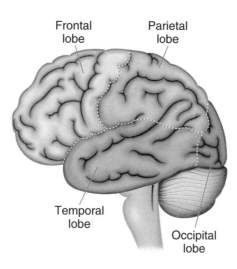

FIGURE 1.3   **Major anatomic divisions of the human brain.**

Reprinted by permission from JH Wilmore and DL Costill, 2004, *Physiology of Sport and Exercise, Third Edition,* (Champaign, IL: Human Kinetics), 69.

about 20 billion. We normally lose an average of 31 million cortical brain cells per year, which is the price we pay for aging. This adds up to an estimated lifetime loss of about 2.5 billion brain neurons (up to about 10% of the total volume of the cortex). This loss is why the brain tends to shrink as we age. Those who abuse alcohol and illegal drugs or who develop certain neurological diseases may experience a greater lifetime loss of brain cells.

The brain is an electrical and chemical organ. It is the cumulative activity of these interrelated electrical and chemical processes that allows us to walk, talk, think, remember, feel, and act. Most of these brain processes are automatic and occur without conscious effort. For example, we don't have to think through every step involved in starting a car and driving it. If we did, we'd take so long that we'd never get anywhere. Perhaps this automatic aspect of behavior is one reason people take the brain for granted.

What Is a Concussion?

Concussion is also known as a traumatic brain injury (TBI) or closed head injury, and about 90% of sport-related concussions are mild in nature and are thus referred to as mild traumatic brain injuries (mTBI). In the general population, closed head injuries (as opposed to *open* head injuries, which involve penetration of the dura, or the covering of the brain under the skull) are classified as mild, moderate, or severe. The severity is typically based initially on a patient's score on the Glasgow Coma Scale (GCS), which is a brief, 3- to 15-point screening scale that assesses eye-opening, motor, and verbal responses. The GCS was developed by Drs. Teasdale and Jennett and was first published in the journal *Lancet* in 1974. Emergency medical technicians and paramedics typically administer the GCS when they arrive at the scene of a head injury. A mild TBI is defined as a GCS score of 13 to 15, a moderate TBI is a GCS score of 9 to 12, and a severe TBI is a GCS score of 8 or less. Various grading systems, which we discuss in chapter 3, have been used for most sport-related concussions.

Head injuries and concussions have been discussed in the medical literature for thousands of years. An excellent article by Drs. Paul McCrory and Samuel Berkovic, published in the journal *Neurology* (2001), summarized the medical history of concussion. Although Hippocrates (460-370 BC) discussed head injuries in his writings, and Galen (2nd century) was probably the first sports medicine physician (as surgeon to the gladiators), the physician Rhazes (9th century) was the first physician to use the term *concussion*. LaFrancus (13th century) viewed concussion as a transient paralysis of cerebral (brain) function caused by the soft brain being shaken against a hard skull (i.e., commotion). The word *concussion* derives from the Latin term *cerebrum commotum*. The effects of concussion were originally conceived as caused by a shaking of the brain.

In sports, concussions have been known in the past as a *ding* (Yarnell and Lynch, 1973) or a *bell-ringer*. Phrases such as "he got his bell rung," "she was shaken up," or "he saw stars" were common descriptors of concussions. A concussion was viewed primarily as a transient, routine event that occurred with regularity during athletic contests and was rarely taken very seriously. In fact, athletes and sports medicine professionals have often shown greater initial concern for an ankle sprain than for a brain sprain (concussion). We have been amazed that in professional sports a sprained ankle or a bruised muscle seemed to warrant an immediate MRI scan whereas a concussed player was urged to "shake it off." Figure 1.4 depicts a concussion in collegiate football. It has only been in the past few years that the word "concussion" has appeared with any regularity in the weekly sports page listings of professional athletes' injuries. Indeed, in 2004 the National Athletic Trainers' Association,

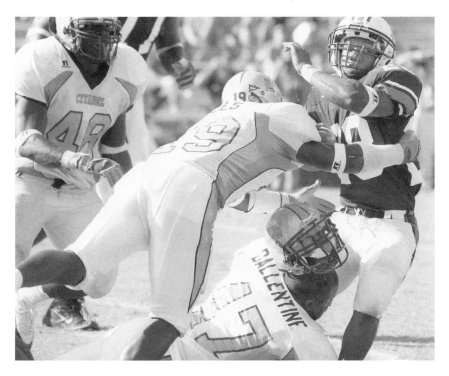

FIGURE 1.4 Note the ball carrier's right knee impacting the defender's head and dislodging his helmet.

Photo by Russ Pace—The Citadel.

in its position paper on sport-related concussion, advocated for the eradication of the colloquial term "ding" when referring to concussion because the term was viewed as diminishing the seriousness of the injury (Guskiewicz et al. 2004).

Numerous definitions of concussion have appeared in the professional literature over the years. In 1966 the Ad Hoc Committee to Study Head Injury Nomenclature of the Congress of Neurological Surgeons defined concussion as "a clinical syndrome characterized by immediate and transient post-traumatic impairment in neural function, such as alteration of consciousness, disturbance of vision, equilibrium, etc. due to brain stem involvement due to mechanical forces" (cited in Maroon et al. 2000, p. 661).

In 1996, the National Football League's Mild Traumatic Brain Injury Committee (Pellman et al. 2003a), in anticipation of their 5-year research project, offered a definition of concussion. Concussion was defined as follows:

. . . For this research, a reportable MTBI was defined as a traumatically induced alteration in brain function, manifested by an alteration of awareness or consciousness, including but not limited to a loss of consciousness, "ding," sensation of being dazed or stunned, sensation of "wooziness" or "fogginess," seizure, or amnestic period, and by symptoms commonly associated with postconcussion syndrome, including persistent headaches, vertigo, light-headedness, loss of balance, unsteadiness, syncope [fainting], near-syncope, cognitive dysfunction, memory disturbances, hearing loss, tinnitus [ringing in the ears], blurred vision, diplopia [double vision], visual loss, personality change, drowsiness, lethargy, fatigue, and inability to perform usual daily activities. (p. 800) (*Note:* bracketed information inserted.)

The American Academy of Neurology (1997) defined concussion as follows:

A trauma-induced alteration in mental status that may or may not involve loss of consciousness. Confusion and amnesia are the hallmarks of concussion. The confusional episode and amnesia may occur immediately after the blow to the head or several minutes later. (p. 582)

In 1999, the American Orthopedic Society for Sports Medicine (Wojtys, et al. 1999) defined concussion this way:

Any alteration in cerebral function caused by a direct or indirect (rotation) force transmitted to the head resulting in one or more of the following acute signs or symptoms: a brief loss of consciousness, light-headedness, vertigo [dizziness], cognitive and memory dysfunction, tinnitus, blurred vision, difficulty concentrating, amnesia, headache, nausea, vomiting, photophobia [sensitivity to light], or a balance disturbance. Delayed signs and symptoms may also include sleep irregularities, fatigue, personality changes, an inability to perform usual daily activities, depression, or lethargy. (p. 676) (*Note:* bracketed information inserted.)

The Concussion in Sport Group (CIS; 2002) defined concussion as follows:

A complex pathophysiological process affecting the brain, induced by traumatic biomechanical forces. Several common features that incorporate clinical, pathological, and biomechanical injury constructs that may be used in defining the nature of concussive head injury include:

1. Concussion may be caused either by a direct blow to the head, face, neck, or elsewhere on the body with an "impulsive" force transmitted to the head.
2. Concussion typically results in the rapid onset of short-lived impairment of neurological function that resolves spontaneously.
3. Concussion may result in neuropathological changes, but the acute clinical symptoms largely reflect a functional disturbance rather than structural injury.
4. Concussion results in a graded set of clinical syndromes that may or may not involve loss of consciousness. Resolution of the clinical and cognitive symptoms typically follows a sequential course.
5. Concussion is typically associated with grossly normal neuroimaging studies.

British Journal of Sports Medicine, 2002, vol. 36, pp. 6-7. Reproduced with permission from the BMJ Publishing Group.

The World Health Organization (WHO) Collaborating Centre for Neurotrauma Task Force on Mild Traumatic Brain Injury proposed a new definition for mTBI in the *Journal of Rehabilitative Medicine* (Carroll et al. 2004). Their definition, which is designed to be used for general use (not necessarily specific to sports), is as follows:

MTBI is an acute brain injury resulting from mechanical energy to the head from external physical forces. Operational criteria include (i) 1 or more of the following: confusion or disorientation, loss of consciousness for 30 minutes or less, post-traumatic amnesia for less than 24 hours, and/or other transient neurological abnormalities such as focal signs, seizure, and intracranial lesion not requiring surgery; (ii) Glasgow Coma Scale score of 13 to 15 after 30 minutes postinjury or later upon presentation for healthcare. These manifestations of MTBI must not be due to drugs, alcohol, medications, caused by other injuries or treatment for other injuries (for example, systemic injuries, facial injuries or **intubation**), caused by other problems (for example, psychological trauma, language barrier or coexisting medical conditions) or caused by penetrating **craniocerebral** injury. (p. 115)

The CIS (2002) definition represents a consensus of thinking from many experts in the sports medicine field and is recommended as most current.

> **intubation**—The insertion of a tube into the throat to assist with breathing.
>
> **craniocerebral**—Pertaining to the cranium (head) and cerebrum (the main portion of the brain containing the two hemispheres).

The progressive lengthening of the definition of concussion over the years attests to the complexity of the phenomena of concussion and highlights the differing medical opinions about it. As you can see, definitions of concussion have been offered over the years by neurosurgeons, neurologists, orthopedic surgeons, and multidisciplinary groups. Although the various definitions are more similar than different, some researchers have viewed the previous lack of agreement about the definition of concussion among professional groups as a barrier to more progress in this important area. With the consensus CIS definition, this lack of agreement may no longer be the case.

Are Head Injuries in Sports Really a Problem?

According to The Centers for Disease Control and Prevention (CDC 1997), there are as many as 300,000 sports-related concussions annually in the United States. This number yields an average of 822 sport concussions per day. Seventy-five percent of these concussions are classified as mild, but 9% of individuals are hospitalized. Among the general population in the United States, the annual incidence of concussion is estimated at 1.54 million (4,219 per day each year). Many believe that this is an underestimation of the incidence of concussion because many milder injuries are undiagnosed or are not brought to medical attention. More important than underreporting is the frightening fact that the injury is most often not even recognized by professional athletes (Delaney et al. 2000).

Studies summarized by Dr. Scott Grindel (2003) indicate that an estimated 900 deaths occur annually in sports and recreation due to an injury to the brain. Unfortunately, brain and spinal cord injuries have occurred routinely in sports for many years. In fact, it was concern about the increasing number of football-related fatalities that led President Theodore Roosevelt to encourage the formation of the National Collegiate Athletic Association (NCAA) in the early 1900s.

The compilation of football-related deaths began in 1931. Doctors Robert Cantu and Frederick Mueller head the National Center for Catastrophic Sports Injury Research, headquartered at the University of North Carolina at Chapel Hill since 1965. These doctors reported in 2003 that 497 injuries to the central nervous system resulted in fatalities in American football between 1945 and 1999. Brain injuries caused 69% of these deaths, cervical-spine (upper-neck) injuries caused 16%, and various other injuries caused 15%. **Subdural hematoma** and **parenchymal hemorrhages** were associated with the majority (429 of 497, or 86%) of the brain-injury-related fatalities. A majority (61%) of the brain-injury-related fatalities occurred during football games; 75% of these fatalities were high school football players. The authors emphasize that the number of high school football players in the United States is over one million, far greater than the estimated number of collegiate (about 75,000) or professional (about 2,000) players. One worrisome finding from these data is that high school football players have the greatest odds of suffering a fatal head injury while playing the game.

> **subdural hematoma**—A localized collection of blood (and spinal fluid) in the space underneath the outer covering of the brain (the dura) usually resulting from a laceration in the brain and/or a tear in a blood vessel.
>
> **parenchymal hemorrhages**—The escape of blood from capillaries in the brain.

The good news is that football fatalities have decreased over the years. In 1950, approximately 30 football players died annually. From 1971 to 1984, the average was about 8 deaths per year (Torg et al. 1985). This average had decreased to an average of about 5 football-related deaths per year by 2001 (Bailes and Cantu 2001). Two factors are presumed responsible for this decrease. First, a 1976 football rule change prohibited initial contact with the head and face when blocking and tackling (a practice known as *spearing*). However, as you will see in chapter 5, spearing still occurs with regularity in professional football. Second, the National Operating Committee on Standards for Athletic Equipment recommended changes that went into effect in 1976 for colleges and 1980 for high schools. These changes improved the protective quality of football equipment (for example, helmet padding and design, and stability of chinstraps). Despite these efforts, however, at least one football-related fatality has occurred in the United States every year from 1945 to 1999, with the sole exception of the year 1990 (Mueller 2001).

Dr. Frederick Mueller (2001) reported that from 1984 to 1999, 69 head-related football injuries resulted in permanent disability. Sixty-three of the 69 injuries (91.3%) were associated with high school football, while the remaining six were in collegiate athletes. Again, high school football players appear to be at the greatest risk for football-related disabilities. Twenty other deaths and 19 permanent disability injuries were reported from 1982 to 1999 in sports other than football, with the greatest proportions in track and field, baseball, and cheerleading. Three deaths and three permanent disabilities have occurred in female athletes.

Drs. Julian Bailes and Robert Cantu (2001) estimated that about 4 to 5 deaths occur each year in the United States as a result of a football-related head injury. Keep in mind, however, that snow skiing leads to about 32 deaths per year, and skateboarding accounts for 7 deaths per year. The recreational sport that accounts for the most deaths per year in the United States is bicycling, with 1,000 to 1,300 estimated deaths annually (half of whom are children and adolescents, with the majority of deaths caused by brain injury). To put this in even sharper perspective (and as we will see in chapter 5), Bailes (2004) estimated that about 1,300 deaths have resulted from the sport of boxing since 1880. This means that more cyclists are killed *every year* than the total sum of boxers who have died in competition in about 125 years of boxing.

In the same article, Bailes and Cantu (renowned neurosurgeons in sports medicine) present some very interesting data on fatalities and catastrophic or serious injuries in U.S. high school and collegiate athletics, which did not include football, for the 15-year period of 1982 through 1997. The total number of fatalities and injuries (catastrophic injuries that typically lead to permanent disability) among high school athletes across all sports (outside football) and seasons during the 15-year period was 138. Track and field led the way with 39, followed by wresting with 33, baseball with 28, gymnastics with 12, and swimming and basketball with 7 each. One death was noted in lacrosse, and none were reported in tennis.

The total number of fatalities and catastrophic injuries among collegiate athletes not including football was 33. Note once again, even when adjusting for relative numbers of athletes, it is the high school athlete who has the greatest risk for a fatal or catastrophic injury—roughly *four* times the risk compared to collegiate athletes. Among the collegiate athletes, mortality (death) and morbidity (permanent disability) were highest in track and field and ice hockey (7 each), followed by gymnastics with 6, baseball and lacrosse with 4 each, basketball with 3, and swimming and wrestling, 1 each. Again, none were reported in tennis.

When we look at the numbers in terms of rate of total direct fatalities and injuries per 100,000 participants (which adjusts the rate for overall number of athletes), the highest risk for high school athletes was in ice hockey and gymnastics. For collegiate athletes, the converse pattern was found, with gymnastics having the highest risk and ice hockey the second highest.

Equestrian sports (horseback riding) are not included in the Bailes and Cantu (2001) data, primarily because these are typically not considered a routine high school or college sport. However, the number of head and neck injuries and fatalities in horseback riding is significant, and safety measures should be used routinely in these activities. For an excellent review of the data on head injury and concussion in equestrian sports, see the chapter by Broshek, Brazil, Freeman, and Barth (2004).

These numbers may appear frightening. However, the numbers tell us that an individual in the United States is much more likely to suffer death or disabling injury from recreational cycling than from any other sport, either at the high school or college levels. So put on your helmet when you ride your bike, and make sure children do as well.

Second-Impact Syndrome

In 1973, neurosurgeon R.C. Schneider (who has been called "the illustrious grandfather of neurosurgical sports medicine" by Dr. Robert Cantu) and his colleagues published a case study of an athlete who died from a second blow to the head before recovering fully from an initial concussion. This phenomenon was later termed *second-impact syndrome of catastrophic head injury* by Drs. R.L. Saunders and R.E. Harbaugh (1984).

Dr. Cantu has defined second-impact syndrome (SIS) as a condition that occurs when an athlete who has sustained a head injury—usually a concussion or cerebral contusion—sustains a second head injury before symptoms associated with the first injury have cleared. The consequences can be lethal. SIS highlights the importance of taking concussion seriously and ensuring that an athlete recovers fully from an initial concussion before being exposed to the potential for another. Because of concern about SIS, the NCAA (1994) adopted guidelines in an attempt to prevent its occurrence. The guidelines were revised in 2002.

In the typical case of SIS, an athlete (usually children, adolescents, or young adults) sustains a concussion and experiences the usual symptoms (headache, concentration problems, feeling slowed down, nausea). Before the resolution of these symptoms, which can take days or a week or more, the athlete returns to competition and sustains a second blow to the head, which may appear rather trivial. The athlete may appear stunned or dazed, much as one would expect after an apparently mild concussion. However, within 15 seconds to minutes after the second impact, the conscious athlete suddenly falls to the ground and becomes comatose, with rapidly dilating pupils, loss of eye movement, and evidence of respiratory failure. The usual time from second impact to brainstem failure (the brainstem controls breathing) is from 2 to 5 minutes. Drs. Bailes and Cantu estimate a SIS mortality rate approaching 50% and a morbidity rate (patients left with disabling conditions) of nearly 100%. Although SIS is relatively rare, 35 cases of probable SIS were identified in American football alone between 1980 and 1993. According to Dr. Joseph Maroon and colleagues (2000), 26 cases of SIS-related deaths have been confirmed in the United States since 1984. Six case studies of SIS (one from hockey and six from boxing) were reported in a 1995 article by Drs. Robert Cantu and Robert Voy in the journal *The Physician and Sportsmedicine*.

What happens in the brain during SIS? The brain is usually very adept at regulating its blood supply (termed **autoregulation**). In SIS, autoregulation is disrupted (as a result of the effects of the concussion), with the result being massive edema (swelling) and raised intracranial pressure. The result of the swelling and pressure is the **herniation** of the brain (a part of the brain protrudes beyond its normal boundaries). In short, the brain expands and no longer fits within the skull, leading to tragic consequences. Cases of SIS are not restricted to boxing or hockey, and SIS has been reported in football players and downhill skiers.

It should be noted that Dr. Paul McCrory (2001b), a leading Australian sports medicine neurologist, has questioned the existence of SIS as a second injury. He proposed that SIS is not a distinct complication of recurrent concussion but is a more basic clinical condition representing diffuse cerebral swelling, a well-known complication of traumatic brain injury (particularly in children and adolescents). Dr. McCrory did not, however, question the potentially lethal complications.

autoregulation—The intrinsic tendency of an organ to maintain constant blood flow despite changes in arterial pressure, thereby providing for its typical metabolic needs.

herniation—The abnormal protrusion of an organ or other body structure through a defect or natural opening in its covering structure.

He and his colleagues (2000) have pointed out that SIS has never been documented in a professional athlete.

Whatever we call it, it is clear to us that no concussed athlete should be allowed to return to play before he or she has had all symptoms completely cleared. This situation appears to be especially important with younger athletes. Although SIS is rare, it is life threatening and therefore should be taken quite seriously. As athletic trainers and sports medicine physicians often say, "When in doubt, sit them out!" This advice is simple but sound.

Increased Awareness for Sport Concussion

The year 2001 may well have been the year for reporting on sport concussion in professional journals. The *Clinical Journal of Sport Medicine* (Volume 11, number 3) and the *Journal of Athletic Training* (Volume 36, number 3) devoted entire issues to sport concussion. The *Journal of Clinical and Experimental Neuropsychology* (Volume 23, number 6) was a special issue addressing "Mild to Moderate Traumatic Brain Injury" (but not specific to athletes). Articles in prominent professional journals such as *Neurosurgery, Journal of Child Neurology,* and *American Family Physician* were sport concussion related. The effect of multiple concussions on the careers of many high-profile professional athletes was a recurrent theme in many newspaper articles and television reports.

Someone unfamiliar with sports in North America might conclude that a sudden epidemic of sports-related concussions occurred in 2001. Nothing could be further from the truth. The truth is that concussions have always existed in sports, but these injuries have generally been viewed as trivial, inconsequential, or insignificant. A search of the professional literature shows that articles have been published since the 1970s on the possibly deleterious effects of sport concussion. Interest in this area grew in the 1980s, and articles began to appear with greater regularity and across various professional disciplines and organizations in the 1990s.

For most athletes, trainers, neuropsychologists, and physicians, 2001 marked the year that many began to take concussion more seriously. As Bailes and Cantu (2001) wrote in *Neurosurgery,*

The current realization that mild traumatic brain injury (MTBI) or concussion represents a major health consideration with more long-ranging effects than previously thought . . . we no longer consider the "dinged" states of athletic concussions to have the benign consequences they had in the past. (p. 26)

Ferrara and associates (2001) surveyed nearly 400 ATCs (who were working with high school, collegiate, and professional athletes) attending the 1999 National Athletic Trainers Association Annual Meeting and Clinical Symposia. At that point in time, ATCs were utilizing clinical evaluation and symptom checklists and collaboration with physicians as the primary strategy for concussion assessment. It was reported that 83.5% of the ATCs believed the following:

> The use of a standardized method of concussion assessment provided more information than routine clinical and physical examination alone . . . athletic trainers are beginning to use standardized methods of concussion to evaluate these injuries and to assist them in assessing the severity of injury and deciding when it is safe to return to play. (p. 145)

As mentioned earlier, articles on sport concussion began appearing with regularity in the professional literature and in the popular press around 2001. For example, in 2001 an article appeared in the journal *Medicine and Science in Sports and Exercise* titled "Concussions in Hockey: There Is Cause for Concern." In 2002, an article appeared in *USA Today* detailing the development of a new football helmet (Riddell's "Revolution") designed to afford greater protection for the head and hopefully reduce the probability and severity of a concussion. Articles related to concussion in NASCAR drivers appeared in *USA Today* in 2002, and the same publication printed an article in 2003 on the efforts made by the NHL to curb concussions in its players. The year 2003 also saw articles in professional journals related to athletes' knowledge about the symptoms of concussion, as well as one study that compared reporting systems for concussion in NCAA Division I football. These examples are only a sampling of the types of information exploding in the literature on sport-related concussion. Those involved in other sports not mentioned here should also be aware of the risk of concussion, as is seen in the wrestling position depicted in figure 1.5.

The increasing importance of and attention to concussion in sports were highlighted in an announcement in the January 2003 issue of the journal *Neurosurgery*. In that issue, Editor Dr. Michael Apuzzo announced the appointment of Dr. Robert Cantu as the principal of the Sports section of the journal. Dr. Cantu, in a letter

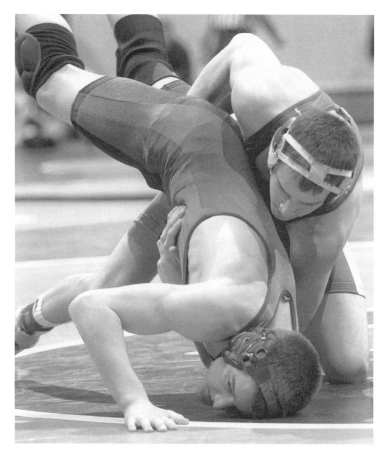

FIGURE 1.5   Concussion in wrestling is a common injury.
© Human Kinetics.

to the readership of the journal, acknowledged the historical contributions of neurosurgeons to sports medicine, but he bemoaned
the fact that neurosurgeons had largely failed to claim their place in
sport concussion. He exhorted his colleagues to take a "prominent
position" in the sports medicine community. We hope they make
the effort to support this need.

In addition to greater awareness of concussion, it is possible
that concussive injury is occurring with greater frequency than
in the past, at least in some sports. For example, Wennberg and
Tator (2003) reported that during the 16 years between 1986 and
2002, the average size of a NHL player increased by one inch (2.54
centimeters) in height and nine pounds (4 kilograms) in weight.
The size of the hockey rink has not been changed. Although we

do not have data on average height and weight of NFL players, we suspect that average player size has increased substantially over time. Once again, the size of the field in the NFL has not changed. It is also plausible to believe that the average NHL or NFL athlete has greater speed and strength than in the past. Increased height, weight, strength, and speed might also be the case for collegiate and high school athletes. Combining the variables of increased mass and velocity in the context of unchanged space, basic physics would suggest greater force and hence the probability of a greater number of concussions.

It is safe to conclude that sport concussion is finally beginning to get the attention it deserves. We would hasten to add, however, that agreement is not uniform among health care professionals or sports coaches and management as to the relative importance or potential significance of sport concussion. We have heard several athletes comment that their coach, trainer, or doctor "doesn't believe" in the potential severity of the consequences of concussion. On many occasions we have heard former athletes say something like, "Well, when I was playing, I got my bell rung a lot and nobody made a big deal about it; you just sucked it up and got back out there." To them I (GS) typically reply, "Well, when I was playing (actually, riding the bench), they wouldn't let us drink water during practices and had us take salt pills all the time." We now know that restricting fluid intake during strenuous exertion is probably one of the worst things an athlete can do. We have learned much over the years; perhaps it's time to update our knowledge base in a variety of areas, including concussion.

We encourage our readers to visit www.HumanKinetics.com/TheHeadsUpOnSportConcussion for a free download of a poster dedicated to concussion education. We developed this poster with the goal of presenting a concise overview of concussion facts, the signs and symptoms of concussion, and treatment recommendations. We hope that sports medicine professionals and families will take advantage of this poster to increase personal and public knowledge about sport-related concussion.

How Many Athletes Get Concussions?

Any athlete is potentially at risk for concussion. We have taken a look at the death and disability data as a result of head injury in high school and collegiate athletes. Now let's look at the published data on concussions in these players.

The incidence of concussion in sports has been a topic of study since the 1980s. Annual rates of concussion in high school and collegiate football players have ranged from a low of 4% (Zariczny et al. 1980) to a high of 7.7% (Barth et al. 1989), with intermediate rates reported in other studies (for example, Guskiewicz et al. 2000; McCrea et al. 1997). Echemendia (1997) surveyed incoming collegiate male freshmen about their cumulative high school concussion history. He found that 55.8% of hockey, 41.2% of soccer, 36.8% of basketball, and 29.8% of football athletes reported having sustained a concussion during their high school career.

Powell and Barber-Foss (1999), in a survey of high school athletes, reported annual concussion rates in women of 4.3% for soccer, 3.6% for basketball, 2.5% for field hockey, and 1% for volleyball. Echemendia (1997), in the study just described, found cumulative concussion rates in incoming female freshmen of 42.2% in soccer and 31.3% in basketball.

Dr. Scott Delaney (2004) reported data estimating the total number of head injuries, concussions, internal head injuries, and skull fractures in the United States for the years 1990 to 1999. These data were based on reports from hospital emergency departments and were compiled for the U.S. Consumer Product Safety Commission using the National Electronic Injury Surveillance System. 68,861 concussions were football related; 21,715 were related to soccer; and 4,820 were ice hockey related. Delaney concluded that although the total numbers of injuries to the head differed among the three sports, the yearly concussion rates were comparable. Keep in mind that these data reflect concussive injuries leading to a visit to the emergency room.

Again, although the numbers are somewhat similar, they differ (at least in part) because of the varying definitions of concussion used by sports medicine professionals, variable diagnostic practices among sports medicine professionals, and the reliance on an athlete's self-report (or self-diagnosis) of concussion, which may not be reliable. The NCAA's Injury Surveillance System tracks data on athletic-related injuries (reported by team ATCs and physicians). From 1984 to 1991, concussions were estimated to account for anywhere from 1.8% to 4.5% of all injuries. From 1995 to 1996, concussions accounted for 1.6% to 6.4% of all injuries. For NCAA men in the 1997 to 1998 season, the relative risk for concussion (per 1,000 athletic exposures, which includes games and practices) was highest in hockey for men and in lacrosse for women. Simply stated, on average, for all genders, sports, and levels of competition (high school or college), based on the data in the previous studies it appears that an athlete's odds of sustaining a reported concussion in any one season is roughly 5%, or 1 in 20.

Unfortunately, research indicates that we may still be underestimating the incidence of concussion in many sports. In 2000, Dr. Scott Delaney and associates reported that four out of five professional football players did not know when they had sustained a concussion. Other studies by Delaney and colleagues (2001, 2002) surveyed collegiate football and soccer players about symptoms of concussion in the prior athletic season. About one-third (34.1%) of the football players and one-half (46.2%) of the soccer players reported having experienced these symptoms during the prior season. Remarkably, however, only one-sixth (16.7%) of the football players and one-third (29.2%) of the soccer players realized that they had suffered a concussion. Delaney concluded, "Despite being relatively common, many players may not recognize the symptoms of a concussion" (2002, p. 1).

Thus, lack of awareness by an athlete of the symptoms of concussion may be a contributing factor to the underestimation of the incidence of concussion. Conscious nonreporting of a concussion may be another factor. Dr. Michael McCrea and his colleagues (2004) administered a confidential survey to varsity football players in Milwaukee, Wisconsin, at the end of a football season. The authors defined concussion as follows:

> A blow to the head followed by a variety of symptoms that may include any of the following: headache, dizziness, loss of balance, blurred vision, "seeing stars," feeling in a fog or slowed down, memory problems, poor concentration, nausea, or throwing up. Getting "knocked out" or being unconscious does NOT always occur with a concussion. (p. 14)

Nearly one-third (29.9%) of the athletes reported having had a concussion prior to this year's season, and 15.3% reported sustaining a concussion during the current football season. Most surprising, however, was the fact that less than half of the players (47.3%) reported their injury. When asked why they did not report the concussion, about two-thirds (66.4%) of the athletes felt the injury was not serious enough to warrant medical attention. About one-third (36.1%) was unaware that they had sustained a concussion. Not wanting to be kept out of play was a reason given by 41% of the athletes for not reporting symptoms of a concussion, and 22% felt that they would be letting down their teammates if they reported the concussion. The numbers do not add up to 100% because athletes were able to give more than one reason for not reporting the concussion.

The authors also inquired in the survey as to whom the athletes reported their concussion. The majority reported the concussion to the athletic trainer (76.7%), followed by their coach (38.8%), parent (35.9%), teammate (27.2%), and others (family physician, other student; 11.7%). No relationship was found between having a history of previous concussion (or number of concussions) and the likelihood of reporting the injury during the season. Again, the numbers do not add up to 100% because athletes may have reported the concussion to more than one source.

The studies by Delaney, McCrea, and their colleagues highlight two possible reasons for the underestimation of concussion in high school and collegiate football and soccer. First, as pointed out by Delaney, athletes may not be aware that they have sustained a concussion. Second, as shown by McCrea, athletes may be aware that they have had a concussion, but for a variety of reasons they may be unwilling to report it.

If we can generalize the results of these studies to athletes in other sports and at similar or higher levels of competition (i.e., professional), then the published data on the incidence of concussion may have seriously underestimated the frequency with which concussion occurs. It may be the case that the odds of an athlete sustaining a concussion during a football season are about 15% and probably higher, with half of those concussions going unreported and thus improperly treated.

There appears to be a general incidence of about a 1 in 20 (5%) chance per season that an athlete will sustain a reported concussion. However, if the findings of Delaney and McCrea are applicable to athletes in other sports and at multiple levels of participation, then these numbers are underestimations of concussion and the risk is possibly three or more times higher. The data of Delaney and McCrea actually point researchers in a different direction for the future. We may need to start looking at the numbers in terms of *reported* concussions, keeping in mind that a sizeable (and yet to be determined) percentage of concussions go unreported. We also need to better educate athletes about the symptoms of concussion and teach them that attempting to play through or with the symptoms isn't always the best way to go when it comes to concussion.

Research Digest

The Bailes and Cantu (2001) study, which assessed the total number of nonfootball fatalities and catastrophic injuries among athletes during the 1982 to 1997 seasons, was based on a sample size of 44,190,168 high school athletes (approximately 36% female), and 46,500,230 collegiate athletes (approximately 64% male). Among high school athletes, the rate of total direct fatalities and injuries per 100,000 was 3.11 for ice hockey and 2.46 for gymnastics. For collegiate athletes, the rates for gymnastics and ice hockey were 17.39 and 11.55 (per 100,000), respectively.

McCrea et al.(1998) found a concussion-incidence rate of 5.5% in high school and collegiate football players. Powell and Barber-Foss (1999) found a 4.7% concussion rate among 21,000 players representing 351 high school teams (across various sports and for both genders). For males, concussions accounted for 7.3% of football, 4.4% of wrestling, 3.9% of soccer, 2.6% of basketball, and 1.7% of baseball injuries. For females, concussion accounted for 4.3% of soccer, 3.6% of basketball, 2.5% of field hockey, and 1.0% of volleyball injuries. For males, Guskiewicz et al. (2000) reported a 5.1% concussion rate among 17,549 high school and collegiate football players.

The NCAA Injury Surveillance System data (1997 to 1998) reported the relative risk per 1,000 athletic exposures (games and practices) for men and women. For women, the rates were 0.62 for lacrosse, 0.58 for soccer, and 0.29 for basketball. For men, the rates were 0.56 for ice hockey, 0.49 for wrestling, 0.43 for football, 0.35 for soccer, and 0.33 for lacrosse.

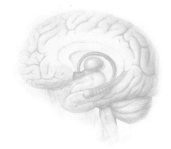

chapter 2

Brain Processes and Symptoms

In this chapter we discuss the physical and chemical changes that occur in the brain during a concussion, review the typical symptoms of a concussion, and discuss the role of loss of consciousness in sport concussion.

What Happens in the Brain During a Concussion?

Let's first take a look at the biomechanical or physical forces that affect the brain. The biomechanical forces can result in microscopic structural changes in the brain, which then lead to changes at the chemical level. As you will see, the type of biomechanical force causing a concussion can have different effects on the features of a concussion, such as loss of consciousness. After we review the biomechanical forces, we will then look at what happens chemically in the brain during and after a concussion.

Biomechanical Forces

In a concussion, biomechanical forces have an impact on the brain directly or indirectly. Two major types of forces occur: (a) acceleration-deceleration (linear) and (b) rotational. In acceleration-deceleration impacts, a force (for example, another player) impacts a player's head and causes acceleration, moving the brain in one direction. The stricken player's head is then eventually stopped by another object (for example, the ground in football or the boards in hockey), which leads to deceleration (stopping the brain from moving in the previous accelerated direction). This biomechanical dynamic is illustrated in figure 2.1.

In rotational impacts, the head is rotated from side to side by an external force. For example, a cross punch in boxing might impact the left side of an opponent's jaw and cause the person's head to move to the right (the side opposite the impact). This type of biomechanical force is depicted in figure 2.2. In both acceleration-deceleration and rotational impacts, nerve cells in the brain (**neurons**) can be stretched and torn. Particularly

> **neurons**—A brain cell, or any cell of the central nervous system. Neurons have a nucleus, a long process that terminates in twiglike branches (axon), and several short radiating processes (dendrites).

1. Brain moves forward in skull.

3. Rebound movement (contre-coup) causes injury to occipital lobe.

2. Frontal lobes strike inside of skull (contusion).

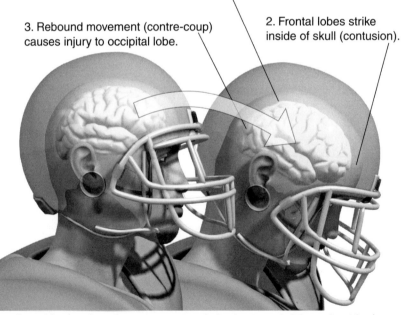

Stretching/tearing of neurons occurs in brain stem and throughout brain.

FIGURE 2.1   Linear forces in concussion.

Redrawn, by permission, from Dr. M. Lovell.

vulnerable is the axon, which is the part of the neuron that interconnects with other nerve cells. Rotational head injuries tend to be more instrumental in sport concussion than linear impacts. A rotational injury is often the cause of a knockout punch in boxing, like the cross punch previously described. A linear impact (that is, a straight-ahead force) almost never results in loss of consciousness. If linear impacts caused loss of consciousness, the floor of the forest would be littered with woodpeckers with self-inflicted concussive injuries. For an excellent and in-depth review of the biomechanics of brain injury in athletes, see the chapter by Newman (2004).

Most sport concussions do not involve gross structural injury to the brain, which is why most **computed axial tomography (CT)** and **magnetic resonance imaging (MRI)** scans of

> **computed axial tomography (CAT, or CT)**—A specialized X-ray technique that allows visualization of detailed areas of the body in a specific plane.
>
> **magnetic resonance imaging (MRI)**—A specialized diagnostic technique that utilizes magnetic, X-ray, and nuclear methods to provide a detailed image of specific body areas.

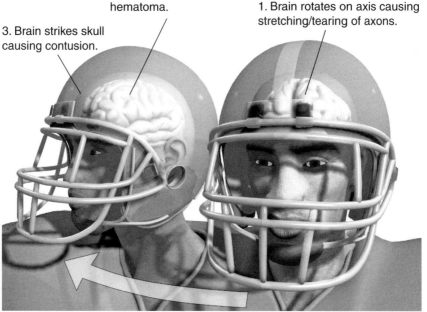

2. Stretching/tearing of blood vessels results in hematoma.

3. Brain strikes skull causing contusion.

1. Brain rotates on axis causing stretching/tearing of axons.

FIGURE 2.2   Rotational forces in concussion.

Redrawn, by permission, from Dr. M. Lovell.

the brain following a concussion are read as normal by the radiologist. However, when structural injuries occur, they are sometimes due to **diffuse axonal injury (DAI),** which involves stretching, compressing, or tearing of the axons that interconnect the cells. DAI is most frequently seen in moderate to severe head injuries. DAI may be rather rare in most sport-related concussions. Some of these lesions in DAI (especially in severe head injury) are observable on CT or MRI scans and are referred to as *shearing injuries.* However, the injury to the brain cells in mild, sport-related concussion is typically not observable on a CT or MRI scan. This is a good example of the old maxim in neurology: "Absence of evidence is not evidence of absence."

Changes in Brain Chemistry During and After a Concussion

Chemical and electrical activities occur in the brain constantly. Figure 2.3 depicts the immediate effects of the "chemical cascade" of concussion. The horizontal axis represents time after concussion (initially in minutes), with the latter part representing days 1 through 10 postconcussion. The vertical axis represents the percentage above normal for each chemical in the cascade. According to Dr. David Hovda (Hovda et al. 1999) and Dr. Chris Giza (Giza and Hovda 2001), the brain **neurotransmitter** glutamate is released immediately (up to 50% above normal) after a concussion. High **glutamate** levels can be toxic to nerve cells. In addition, potassium exits brain cells at up to 400% of normal rate (the second highest line in figure 2.3). Unconsciousness occurs when the potassium level exceeds a critical concentration and the normal electrical processes in the brain (the "action potential," which is necessary for brain cells to communicate) are disrupted. Calcium (depicted by the highest spiking line in figure 2.3) then enters the brain cells at up to 500% of the normal rate. Calcium has an intimate effect on blood flow in the brain. Blood flow in the brain

diffuse axonal injury (DAI)— Widespread injury to the axons of the brain, which are the projections that interconnect nerve cells. Axons are sheared and torn, stretched, or compressed, usually as a result of trauma to the head. DAI disrupts cognitive and neurological function. The lesions are typically visible only at a microscopic level.

neurotransmitter—A naturally occurring substance in the brain that serves as a chemical messenger from one nerve cell to the next. Neurotransmitters allow neurons to communicate and serve as the biological basis for cognitive functioning.

glutamate—A neurotransmitter in the brain.

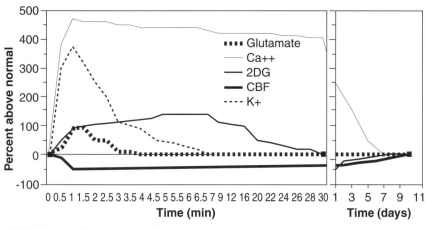

FIGURE 2.3   Chemical cascade of concussion.

Reprinted, by permission, from D.A. Hovda et al., 1999, Neurobiology of concussion. In Sports-related concussion, edited by J.E. Bailes, M.R. Lovell, and J.C. Maroon (St. Louis: Quality Medical Publishing).

(depicted by the line going below 0 in figure 2.3) then decreases up to 50% within 2 minutes of the concussive impact, possibly due to the disruption of the normal calcium processes. The restoration of normal glutamate levels occurs within 3.5 minutes, whereas potassium levels may not return to normal for 20 minutes. Note that calcium levels may not return to baseline for more than 3 days, and blood-flow levels are not restored to normal until a week or so postconcussion.

Along with this chemical cascade, the brain begins to work overtime (a state known as **hypermetabolism**) trying to restore a chemical balance. This results in what Hovda and Giza have termed an "energy crisis." The brain is working hard to restore chemical balance, but there is less oxygen and glucose (brain fuels) to use as an energy source because blood flow in the brain is reduced. It's like trying to catch the lead car on the last lap of a NASCAR race with less than half the normal flow of gas to the engine. Aspects of hypermetabolism can last a day or more.

The brain then enters a state of **hypometabolism** (decreased functioning, often called "resting depression"), which can last 5 to 10-plus days, until blood flow levels in the brain are returned to normal (restored autoregulation of

hypermetabolism—Distinctly increased activity in the physical and chemical processes by which the body produces, maintains, and transforms energy.

hypometabolism—Distinctly decreased activity in the physical and chemical processes by which the body produces, maintains, and transforms energy.

brain's electrochemical and blood-flow processes). This appears to be the time when the brain heals itself. For a more thorough discussion of the abnormalities of biochemistry in traumatic brain injury, see Giza and Hovda (2004).

Can we measure these chemical processes easily and directly? Unfortunately, the answer is no. However, newer research from Europe indicates that several peripheral blood markers of central nervous system activity may be helpful in identifying the severity and outcome probability of brain injury, particularly in *severe* head injuries. These biomarkers include the glial proteins GFAP (glial Fibrillary acidic protein) and S-100B and neuron-specific enolase (NSE).

Vos and colleagues (2004) assessed these biomarkers in 85 patients with *severe* traumatic brain injury (TBI) (not sport related). They found elevated levels of all three biomarkers in the patients with TBI, ranging from 2 to 18 times the normal reference values. Levels of the three biomarkers were significantly elevated in those patients who had died or had a poorer outcome at 6 months (outcome was measured by the Glasgow Outcome Scale) than in those who were alive or had a good outcome. With regard to the use of these measures in mild athletic TBI, Stalnacke and colleagues (2003) reported a pilot study of the effects of playing ice hockey and basketball on serum levels of S-100B and NSE. The authors suggested that S-100B levels might ultimately serve as a biological marker for return-to-play decisions in athletes with concussions. Another pilot Swedish study (Stalnacke et al. 2004) analyzed serum markers of S-100B and NSE in elite soccer players pre- and post-single game competition. The authors also assessed the number of headers (purposely striking the ball with the head) and other trauma events during the game. Both S-100B and NSE levels were elevated after competition compared to pregame values. Number of headers and other trauma events were positively correlated with increases in serum levels of S-100B.

New studies using specialized imaging to measure brain activity are leading to important new findings in concussion. Traditional MRI shows us structure, or what the brain looks like. Although seeing brain structure is quite helpful, it doesn't tell us how the brain is functioning. Remember, the fuels for the brain are oxygen and glucose. Functional MRI indirectly measures oxygen utilization in the brain, showing us where active parts of the brain are working. Functional MRI (fMRI) allows simultaneous cognitive testing and brain imaging and yields a picture similar to the color Doppler radar images we see on television weather reports, with active areas appearing in certain colors. In one study, Chen and colleagues (2004) found concussed athletes who continue to have concussion symptoms have abnormalities in an area of the frontal lobes (particularly in the mid-dorsolateral area of the prefrontal cortex) on fMRI testing. These abnormalities resolve as recovery occurs. Functional MRI testing is one of the first brain-imaging tests to measure concussion injury and recovery.

What can we do to treat the altered electrical and chemical processes in the brain after a concussion? Unfortunately, there is no "PowerAde" for the brain; and, as Mike Tomczak, a retired NFL quarterback said, "There is no way to ice the brain" (Bailes et al. 1999). No drug treatment for concussion is FDA approved at present. For now, the only available treatment is rest, rehabilitation, and the prevention of another concussion.

To say the least, a host of chemical processes are ongoing in the brain during and after a concussion. For most athletes, going through a concussion is a strange time. They are not bandaged, are not limping or bleeding, don't have on a cast, are not walking with crutches, and do not appear to be bruised. Bloom and associates (2004) referred to concussion as an "invisible injury." In short, the athlete has none of the typical external signs or badges worn when injured. They look fine. To conclude that all is well could be a serious mistake. Just because you can't see the injury doesn't mean it's not there.

What Are the Typical Symptoms of Concussion?

Some of the more common symptoms of concussion include headache, nausea, vomiting, balance problems, dizziness, fatigue, sleep disturbance, drowsiness, sensitivity to light and noise, irritability, sadness, nervousness, feeling more emotional, feeling slowed down, feeling mentally foggy, trouble concentrating, feeling pressure in the head, memory dysfunction, and numbness or tingling. It should be noted that this is not an exhaustive or exclusive list. It is important to remember that these symptoms are commonly found in daily life as well as in many medical conditions. In this context, McCrory and Johnston (2002) wrote that the only concussive symptoms that have been validated scientifically were loss of consciousness, headache, dizziness, nausea, blurred vision, memory loss, and difficulty with attention. However, when considering the background of an athlete playing a contact sport, a high index of suspicion for these symptoms is always warranted; and medical evaluation, with careful history taking, is extremely important.

Athletes who have sustained a concussion often have a glazed look, or a befuddled facial expression. The athlete may seem confused, disoriented, and unsure of what to do. She may appear distractible and unable to focus her attention. Speech may be slurred or incoherent. Trouble with gross-motor coordination can be seen, including stumbling and an inability to walk a straight line. Memory deficits may appear in the form of repeating the same question over and over. Emotions may appear inappropriate, such as crying for no apparent reason or displaying emotions out of proportion to the circumstances. Dr. Karen Johnston and colleagues have measured depressive symptoms as a component of concussion in athletes and found them to be common (2004).

Several concussion-symptom checklists are available for use with athletes, and they offer an excellent review of some of the most common symptoms of concussion. Perhaps the best known is the Post-Concussion Scale-Revised (PCS-R), authored by Dr. Mark Lovell and his colleagues. The scale includes 21 common symptoms of concussion. Athletes are instructed to rate each symptom on a 0 to 6 scale, with 0 representing absence of the symptom, 1 to 2 representing a mild level of symptom intensity, 3 to 4 a moderate level, and 5 to 6 a severe level. The PCS-R has been translated into French, Finnish, Russian, and Czech for use in the National Hockey League and other international settings.

Jared Bruce and Dr. Ruben Echemendia published an exploratory-factor analysis of the PCS-R in the journal *Neurology* (2004). Three factors emerged in the analysis. The first factor was labeled "cognitive and balance problems" and included symptoms such as feeling foggy, trouble with balance, and poor concentration. The second factor was termed "sensory and physical symptoms" and included nausea, sensitivity to light and noise, and drowsiness. The third factor was called "emotional disturbance" and included symptoms of irritability, nervousness, and sadness.

Ideally, an athlete would complete the PCS-R prior to beginning a season to obtain a baseline level of symptoms (which is rarely zero) and would complete the scale again postconcussion for comparative purposes. The scale is still useful, however, even if a baseline was not obtained, as it is an excellent review of concussion symptoms. It can be repeated as needed to track resolution of symptoms over time.

A more recent entry in the concussion-symptom checklists is the Head Injury Scale (HIS), introduced in 2003 by Scott Piland, ATC, and colleagues. Piland and his collaborators published a study of the HIS (Piland et al. 2003), which was validated on collegiate (and predominantly male) athletes. The HIS is quite similar to the PCS-R just described.

In addition to the symptoms already noted, concussed players may lose memory of some events that occurred prior to the impact (known as *retrograde* amnesia), whereas others may lose memory of events that occurred after the impact (known as *anterograde* amnesia). It is possible to suffer both retrograde and anterograde amnesia in a concussion. A common misconception among health care professionals is that loss of consciousness (LOC) is necessary in order to experience a concussion. This is not true. As we will see in the next section, most sport-related concussions do not involve LOC. Nor is LOC required to experience retrograde amnesia, anterograde amnesia, or both. Current research suggests that postconcussion symptoms and concussion-related amnesia may be more valuable prognostic signs than LOC (see further discussion on page 35).

A study by Dr. Grant Iverson and colleagues (2004) suggests that the clinical symptom of fogginess may be especially important post-concussion. The authors studied 110 high school athletes who had sustained a sport-related concussion. Athletes rated the presence of fogginess (and other typical postconcussion symptoms) on a 0 to 6 scale and were divided into two groups: 91 with no fogginess and 19 with fogginess. Five to 10 days postconcussion the athletes took a computer-based platform of neuropsychological tests. The athletes with persistent fogginess experienced more concussion-related symptoms and scored more poorly on measures of memory, reaction time, and speed of information processing than the athletes who did not report fogginess.

In our experience, most athletes report headache, dizziness, pressure in the head, and a general comment to the effect of "I just don't feel right" after a concussion. We have come to realize, however, that some athletes seem to have certain constellations of symptoms with their concussion and not others. This observation raises the possibility of concussion subtypes as well as whether particular individuals are more prone or vulnerable to specific postconcussion symptoms than others. This question is an avenue for future research.

Sports medicine professionals who deal with concussions will tell you that many athletes minimize or underreport symptoms after a concussion. This is one reason that neuropsychological testing is important. It's much harder for an athlete to fool the neuropsychological tests than it is for the athlete to just say, "I'm fine."

What is the Role of Loss of Consciousness in Sport Concussion?

Historically, LOC has been viewed by many health care professionals as a necessary condition for the diagnosis of concussion. This is clearly no longer the case, as evidenced by more recent definitions of concussion. Most concussion grading scales have given primary importance to LOC, rating those concussions involving LOC as the most severe. Indeed, most sport-related concussions do not involve LOC. Guskiewicz and colleagues (2000) reported that only 9% of high school and collegiate concussions involve LOC. The very same percentage has been reported among NFL athletes, and the NCAA concussion studies showed about 6% with LOC (see chapter 3). Although LOC should be taken seriously (and may be a precursor of significant medical, cognitive, and neurobehavioral consequences), it is now clear that brief LOC may not be as critical as previously thought.

First, LOC occurs on a time continuum. Part of the problem is that LOC has been viewed as a dichotomous ("yes" or "no," "present" or "absent") variable that does not take into account the amount of time spent unconscious. Therefore, LOC does not account for intermediate states or shades of gray. For example, is LOC of 10 seconds as severe as LOC of 10 minutes? What about a LOC of 24 hours? Is that worse than 10 hours? Is there a specific time window, like 10 minutes, that separates favorable from poor recovery when an athlete suffers LOC? Although intuitively the answer would seem obvious, the fact is we really don't know with certainty.

The American Congress of Rehabilitative Medicine (1993) concluded that LOC lasting longer than 30 minutes was indicative of a more serious form of brain injury than the more routine types of concussion. In the general population, most studies have shown that the length of confusion after a head injury (referred to as "posttraumatic amnesia") is often a better predictor of outcome (recovery) than the length of LOC. Neurologist James Kelly (2001) recommended that sport concussion involving LOC of several minutes should be viewed as a potential neurosurgical emergency requiring urgent medical evaluation. Dr. Kelly concluded that concussion with LOC might be a more serious condition than concussion without LOC but that individual recovery rate was quite variable.

Dr. Mark Lovell and colleagues (1999) addressed the relevance of LOC in predicting neuropsychological test performance in adults with mild head injuries. Patients from a major Pittsburgh hospital served as subjects in the study and were grouped according to LOC (usually less than one minute), no LOC, or uncertain LOC. All patients (383 patients) underwent a series of neuropsychological tests. No significant group differences were found among the three groups on any of the neuropsychological test scores, with all three groups showing "mildly decreased performance" on the tests. The authors concluded, "The results of this study cast doubt on the importance of LOC as a predictor of neuropsychological test performance during the acute phase of recovery from mild traumatic brain injury" (p. 193).

Conversely, Dr. Michael McCrea and colleagues (2002) used the Standardized Assessment of Concussion (SAC) to assess high school and collegiate football players immediately, 15 minutes later, and 48 hours after a concussion. See chapter 3 for a more detailed description of the SAC. Players in the study were grouped as follows: (a) LOC, (b) no LOC, and (c) no LOC but positive posttraumatic amnesia. They found that those players whose concussions involved LOC performed more poorly on the SAC immediately and 15 minutes after a concussion than those with no LOC or brief posttraumatic amnesia. However, scores of all groups on the SAC were equal by 48 hours postconcussion.

Dr. Michael Collins and his collaborators (2003a) studied the relationship between postconcussion headache and neuropsychological test performance in high school athletes. LOC was not associated with the persistence of headache 7 days after the concussion. However, anterograde amnesia was correlated significantly with persistent headache, raising the question of amnesia, as opposed to LOC, as a marker of sport-concussion severity.

Dr. David Erlanger and associates (2003) reported in the *Journal of Neurosurgery* the results of a study of 47 high school, collegiate, and "sports-organizations" athletes who sustained a concussion. Athletes were evaluated with a Web-based neurocognitive test (Concussion Resolution Index) until their results returned to individual baseline levels. The authors found that although LOC was a useful indicator of the initial severity of the injury, it did not correlate with other indices of concussion severity. In particular, LOC did not correlate with duration of concussion symptoms or the overall number of symptoms experienced.

Dr. Mark Lovell and colleagues (2002) studied 160 high school and collegiate athletes with a computer-based neurocognitive measure (called ImPACT; see page 50) preseason and 24 to 48 hours postconcussion. The athletes were divided into LOC and no-LOC groups. No significant differences between groups were observed on the ImPACT Memory, Reaction Time, and Processing Speed Composite scores postconcussion. The authors concluded, "This study supports earlier research that has failed to support the use of LOC as a pre-eminent marker for concussion severity" (p. S-11).

Finally, as we will see when we discuss grading systems for concussion, LOC is receiving less prominence in assessing concussion severity than it did in the past. Again, that is not to say that LOC is not important but that it does not appear to be the critical variable it was once thought to be. Other markers of concussion are emerging as potential predictors of concussion severity, such as the fogginess discussed earlier in the Iverson study (Iverson et al. 2004). Dr. Chad Asplund and associates studied concussion symptoms among 101 athletes across 18 primary care sports medicine sites (91 male athletes, more than half collegiate athletes, representing 6 different sports). The authors found that delayed return to play (defined as greater than 7 days) occurred when concussive symptoms included headache or concentration difficulty lasting more than 3 hours or any retrograde amnesia or LOC.

In short, LOC in sport-related concussion is a condition that may require immediate medical attention in order to rule out an emergency medical condition. However, LOC does not appear to be as crucial as previously thought in the eventual outcome (recovery) from sport concussion. LOC has received less prominence in the more recent grading scales for concussion.

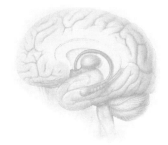

chapter 3

Assessment and Evaluation

This chapter discusses the clinical assessment and evaluation of concussion, including sideline assessment, neuroimaging, neuropsychological testing, balance testing, grading scales (including those of Dr. Robert Cantu and the American Academy of Neurology, which are the two most popular scales), and recovery from concussion.

Many tools exist for the clinical assessment and evaluation of sport concussion. We have divided these tools into the following five basic categories, which we discuss next:

1. Clinical history
2. Sideline-assessment strategies
3. Balance testing
4. Neuroimaging techniques
5. Neuropsychological testing

Clinical History

The first days of training camp typically involve athletes undergoing medical, orthopedic, dental, and vision examinations. Preseason medical evaluation should now routinely include a concussion assessment in which key features of an athlete's history are determined and a complete concussion history is taken (Johnston, Lassonde, Ptito 2001). As an example, details of previous sport and nonsport concussions and injuries (including facial fractures and head injuries) should be collected. Details of the position played by the athlete, protective equipment worn, and attitude as a player may all contribute to understanding a particular athlete's condition.

Guskiewicz and colleagues (2004) emphasize the need for a thorough documented history on athletes with a report of multiple concussions. In particular, they focus on the need to clarify any pattern of concussions occurring as a result of lighter impacts, concussions occurring close in time, a lengthier postconcussion recovery time, and a less complete recovery with each concussion. These factors may point toward a high-risk profile.

Sideline-Assessment Strategies

The sideline assessment of concussion can be approached either qualitatively or quantitatively. A frequently used qualitative measure is Maddocks' Questions. A recommended quantitative measure is the Standardized Assessment of Concussion (SAC). A third measure is the McGill Abbreviated Concussion Evaluation (McGill ACE), which is a hybrid of the two approaches.

In the past, amateur sports teams typically didn't have physicians, athletic trainers, and neuropsychologists available on the sidelines. In most cases (especially in high school), the team coach also served as physician and trainer. Teams were considered especially fortunate if a player's parent was a physician and happened to be a spectator at the game. The typical scenario that occurred when an athlete sustained a concussion was for the coach to place his fist with three fingers extended in front of the athlete's face and ask, "How many fingers?" If the athlete answered correctly, then he was deemed to be okay ("He just got his bell rung") and was allowed to return to play. A more sophisticated approach involved asking the player her name, the date, and where she was. These are basic orientation questions taken from the mental-status examination used in clinical neurology and psychiatry. If the player was able to answer most of these questions correctly, he was assessed as having a "ding" and usually allowed to return to play. Retired NFL players tell stories of passing these screening tests for concussion, returning to play for the rest of the game, and then having no memory whatsoever of what happened in the game.

We now know that such simplistic tasks are inadequate screening measures for assessing sport concussion. The application of traditional clinical mental-status questions and tasks to the evaluation of sport concussion has been woefully inadequate. It is now known that basic orientation questions (such as "What's your name? Where are we? What day is it?") are insensitive to the task of screening for sport concussion. Loss of ability to recall one's name is an extremely rare phenomenon, occurring for example in certain types of psychologically based memory loss (a condition known as "psychogenic amnesia") and in brain diseases such as advanced Alzheimer's disease. Asking a professional athlete for the specific date is usually of little diagnostic value, as athletes are notoriously poor in keeping up with the date. Asking a football player the day of the week also is of little use because high school athletes typically play on Friday nights, collegiate athletes play on Saturdays, and professional athletes typically have games on Sunday.

Maddocks' Questions

To screen players for sport concussion more adequately, a set of orientation questions that reliably differentiated concussed from nonconcussed athletes was needed. Dr. D.L. Maddocks and colleagues provided a solution in 1995 by developing a set of standardized questions that have become known as "Maddocks' Questions":

Which ground (field) are we at?

Which team are we playing today?

Who is your opponent at present?

Which quarter (period) is it?

How far into the quarter (period) is it?

Which side scored the last goal (points)?

Which team did we play last week?

Did we win last week?

Questions should be adapted of course for the specific sport. Maddocks' Questions are a *qualitative* measure for the screening of mental-status abnormalities and are a useful starting point in the initial screening for sport concussion. An athlete's inability to answer Maddocks' Questions correctly should raise suspicion for the presence of a concussive injury and indicates the need for a more thorough assessment.

Standardized Assessment of Concussion

A *quantitative* approach to the sideline assessment of sport concussion was developed by Dr. Michael McCrea and colleagues (1998) when they introduced the Standardized Assessment of Concussion (SAC). The SAC was designed in response to and in accordance with the American Academy of Neurology's practice parameter for concussion (1997), which was an outgrowth of the 1991 Colorado guidelines for the management of concussion in sports. The SAC was also designed based on the available neuropsychological literature demonstrating the domains of brain functioning most sensitive to concussion and the tests best suited to measuring those capacities in patients with brain injuries.

The SAC includes brief measures of orientation, concentration, immediate memory, and delayed recall. The assessment takes about 5 to 6 minutes to administer. The maximum possible score on the SAC is 30 points. Three alternative forms (A, B, and C) are provided for repeat testing as needed. The SAC also includes a standard, brief neurological screening assessing strength, coordination, sensation, and the presence of amnesia. Exertional maneuvers (including sit-ups, knee bends) that are capable of provoking symptoms of concussion also are included in the SAC.

The recommended strategy is to obtain a preseason baseline SAC score on each athlete and then to repeat the SAC on the sideline when an athlete is suspected of having sustained a concussion. Postconcussion SAC scores can then be compared to baseline scores to assess for any possible adverse cognitive effects of the presumed concussion. McCrea's group has shown in published papers that SAC scores are equivalent when the test is given in practice or game conditions and that it is equally effective for discriminating concussed from nonconcussed high school and collegiate athletes. Recent work by McCrea's group (Barr and McCrea 2001) has shown that a 1-point drop between an athlete's postconcussion and baseline performance on the SAC accurately identified 94% of a group of concussed athletes.

Dr. McCrea routinely points out that the SAC is not intended to be a substitute for a neurological examination or for formal neuro-psychological testing. He further notes that return-to-play decisions should not be made on the basis of SAC scores alone. He emphasizes that the SAC is a screening instrument for use on the sidelines. An updated version of the SAC was published in 2000.

McGill Abbreviated Concussion Evaluation

The McGill On-Field Concussion Evaluation, also known as the McGill Abbreviated Concussion Evaluation (ACE), was developed at the McGill Sport Medicine Clinic in Montreal, Quebec, Canada. The ACE is very similar to the SAC and is administered preseason to obtain a baseline and on the field after a possible concussion. It takes about 5 to 10 minutes to complete. The McGill ACE includes immediate memory, concentration, and delayed memory tasks, along with the structured assessment of orientation (including some of Maddocks' Questions), amnesia, and concussion symptoms. Neurological screening and provocative tests of exertion also are included. The orientation, concentration, immediate and delayed memory recall, and amnesia questions are scored quantitatively, with a separate quantitative scoring of concussion symptoms. The McGill ACE has been incorporated into the overall McGill Concussion Protocol.

The McGill ACE has been adapted for use rinkside by team physicians in the National Hockey League (NHL), who complete it on every player suspected of having sustained a concussion during a NHL game.

Other Sideline-Assessment Tools

The University of Pittsburgh Medical Center's Sports Concussion program has published a "Concussion Card" for sideline use. This assessment is a brief mental-status exam for use immediately following concussion. It is essentially a qualitative screening tool that assists the clinician in determining the presence of a concussive injury and is similar to Maddocks' Questions. This brief mental-status exam has been incorporated into Sideline ImPACT, which became available in 2004. Many other clinical sideline aids are available through various sporting organizations, both general and sport specific.

The most recent addition to the armamentarium of sideline-assessment tools is the Sport Concussion Assessment Tool (SCAT). The SCAT was produced as part of the Summary and Agreement Statement of the Second International Symposium on Concussion in Sport held in Prague in 2004. The SCAT is a compilation and condensation of existing instruments that is completed by the sports medicine professional and the athlete. It includes a concussion-symptom checklist, concentration and memory tasks, and neurological screening. The SCAT was published in the April 2005 editions of the *Clinical Journal of Sport Medicine, The Physician and Sportsmedicine,* and the *British Journal of Sports Medicine.*

When choosing which of these assessments to use, it is best to go with what's most comfortable for you. Using Maddocks' Questions is the quickest approach, but it likely has the highest risk (of the approaches described here) of missing a symptomatic athlete. The McGill ACE is probably superior to the SAC in terms of covering concussion *symptoms* in a systematic fashion. The SAC and McGill ACE are otherwise probably equal in the assessment of neurological functions and cognitive domains. The SAC clearly has the upper hand on the McGill ACE in terms of published research supporting its use. We are optimistic about the SCAT and eagerly await published studies on its usefulness. In our opinion, all are superior to the nonstandardized concussion-assessment strategies. What may be more important than the specific test used is the systematic use and application of a valid and reliable strategy that will ensure the adequate assessment of an athlete's concussive symptoms and assist in making diagnostic and return-to-play decisions. See appendix B for information on how to obtain these instruments.

Balance Testing

It is very common for a concussed athlete to complain of problems with dizziness and balance, motor skills that are highly developed in elite athletes. Since the late 1990s, Dr. Kevin Guskiewicz and colleagues have been investigating the use of balance-testing systems in the evaluation of concussed athletes. This approach is a systematic extension of the use of the Romberg test of postural stability, a screening test used routinely in the basic neurological examination in clinical medicine. Guskiewicz (2003) provides an excellent review of the various types of postural-stability tests utilized in the assessment of sport concussion. Clinical balance tests have identified postural-stability deficits lasting several days after a sport-related concussion.

Perhaps the best known and most frequently used system for postural-stability assessment is the Balance Error Scoring System (BESS; Guskiewicz 2001). According to McCrea et al. (2003), the BESS is a noninstrumented clinical assessment of postural stability carried out in single-leg, double-leg, and tandem stances on both firm and foam surfaces. The total score is based on the number of errors made by the athlete, with higher scores representing worse postural stability.

This addition to the assessment of sport concussion may hold promise because initial data have suggested that there appears to be little relationship between **neurocognitive** test scores and postural stability during the very early phases of recovery (Ross et al. 2000). Furthermore, in the National Collegiate Athletic Association (NCAA) football study (McCrea et al. 2003) it was found that balance deficits were most pronounced during the first 24 hours postconcussion but generally resolved by day 5. (See page 56 for more discussion.) The recovery curves indicated that postural-stability deficits resolved slightly earlier than neurocognitive impairments and clinical symptoms. Conversely, Dr. Connie Peterson's (Peterson et al. 2003) prospective study of postural stability and neurocognitive functioning in concussed Division I NCAA athletes found significant differences in composite balance measures and speed of information processing through day 10 postinjury for the concussed athletes when compared to the control group.

As Dr. Kevin Guskiewicz (2001) has observed, the evaluation of postural stability may well be one piece of the puzzle in the assessment of concussion. The National Athletic Trainers' Association (NATA) position statement on sport-related concussion (Guskiewicz et al. 2004) strongly recommended the use of balance testing as part of the baseline and postconcussion assessments. We await further studies on the use of postural-stability assessment in the evaluation of the motor domain of neurological functioning in sport concussion. Plotting recovery curves of postural stability, clinical symptoms, and neurocognitive functions also will be of clinical interest and utility.

neurocognitive—The operations of the mind through which we perceive, think, and remember.

Neuroimaging Techniques

neuroimaging—The applica-
tion of various types of X-ray
and nuclear methods to produce
radiographs (images) of the central nervous system. Computed
tomography (CT) and magnetic
resonance imaging (MRI) are
the most common neuroimaging
methods.

Neuroimaging scans of the brain can be classified as either structural or functional. Structural measures of brain functioning (CT scans and MRI scans) are usually normal after concussion and are not always needed. Structural brain scans are important after some concussions in that they are used to rule out the presence of a brain bleed or other emergency medical condition requiring the intervention and expertise of a neurosurgeon. Structural brain imaging, as opposed to functional measures, is much more commonly used at present in the clinical evaluation of sport-related concussion.

Functional imaging measures of brain activity include functional MRI (fMRI), which indirectly measures oxygen utilization; positron emission tomography (PET), which measures glucose utilization; and single photon emission computed tomography (SPECT), which measures blood flow in the brain. Functional measures of brain functioning are more likely to be abnormal after concussion, as they are measuring the functional processes underlying brain structures. For example, fMRI assesses oxygen utilization in various brain areas during specific tasks. Activated areas are displayed by color, much like color Doppler radar seen on television weather reports. If a subject in a fMRI machine were instructed to listen to spoken words, the picture in figure 3.1 would emerge. Note the activation in the auditory cortex areas.

Conversely, if the subject in the fMRI were asked to look at written words, the image shown in figure 3.2 would emerge, reflecting different areas of brain activation. Note the activation in areas of the visual cortex.

Next, if we ask a subject in a fMRI experiment to speak words, the pattern noted in figure 3.3 emerges. Note the activation of frontal and temporal areas.

Finally, if we asked a subject in a fMRI paradigm to simply think about words, we might see the type of activation pattern and image depicted in figure 3.4. Here we see activation of the frontal and visual areas of the brain.

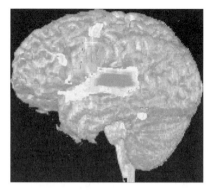

FIGURE 3.1   fMRI of a subject hearing spoken words. Areas in the auditory cortex are activated.

Courtesy of the Alzheimer's Disease Education and Referral Center, a service of the National Institute on Aging.

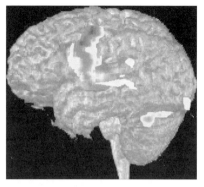

FIGURE 3.2   fMRI of a subject seeing words. Areas in the visual cortex are activated.

Courtesy of the Alzheimer's Disease Education and Referral Center, a service of the National Institute on Aging.

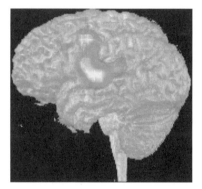

FIGURE 3.3   fMRI of a subject speaking words. Frontal and temporal areas are activated.

Courtesy of the Alzheimer's Disease Education and Referral Center, a service of the National Institute on Aging.

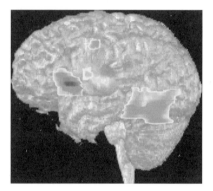

FIGURE 3.4   fMRI of a subject thinking about words. Frontal and visual areas of the brain are activated.

Courtesy of the Alzheimer's Disease Education and Referral Center, a service of the National Institute on Aging.

New fMRI work is ongoing through a National Institute of Health grant to the University of Pittsburgh's Sport Concussion Program. The top scan in figure 3.5 depicts the fMRI scan of a concussed high school athlete 5 days postconcussion. This athlete did not lose consciousness during the concussion. The bottom scan was taken 20 days after the top one. Figure 3.6 depicts the fMRI scans of a control athlete (tennis player) taken at the same times as those of the concussed athlete. Both athletes are performing a working memory task during the fMRI procedure.

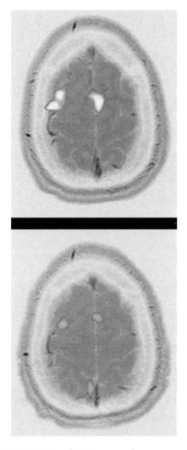

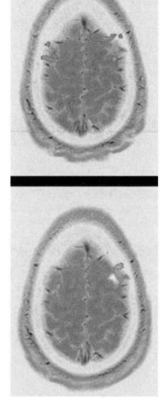

FIGURE 3.5   fMRI scans of a concussed
athlete taken at 5 days postconcussion (top)
and 25 days postconcussion (bottom).

Courtesy of Dr. Mark Lovell.

FIGURE 3.6   fMRI scans of a control
athlete at 5 (top) and 25 (bottom) days
postconcussion.

Courtesy of Dr. Mark Lovell.

In comparing the top scans in both figure 3.5 and figure 3.6 (taken
5 days postconcussion), note the abnormal areas of brain activation (indicating higher oxygen utilization) in the concussed athlete
(top image in figure 3.5). The areas of activation in the dorsolateral
prefrontal cortex noted in the control athlete (top image in figure
3.6) are considered normal for the working memory task being
performed. Both bottom fMRI images were taken 20 days later.
Note how the activation patterns are now more similar between
the control and concussed athletes. In particular, note how the
previous hot activation areas in the concussed athlete (top scan in
figure 3.5) have cooled down (bottom image in figure 3.5).

Similar work with fMRI (Johnston et al. 2001a; Chen et al. 2004) emphasizes the importance of concussion symptoms and reveals abnormalities in brain function (detected on fMRI) that appear to correlate with the duration of symptoms. In other words, the areas of abnormal brain activation tend to dissipate and return to normal as the concussion symptoms resolve. Figure 3.7 depicts these findings.

Dr. Charles Tegeler, Professor of Neurology at the Wake Forest University School of Medicine, has begun to investigate the utility of transcranial Doppler ultrasound (TCD) in the evaluation of sport-related concussion (2004). Dr. Tegeler has employed dynamic vascular analysis to assess the circulatory status of the brain postconcussion. He refers to TCD as the "neurology stethoscope for the brain." His preliminary data have suggested that abnormalities noted on TCD after a concussion may persist even after neurocognitive functions have returned to baseline.

Most functional brain-imaging tests, however, are not used routinely in the clinical assessment of concussion. The reason for not using these tests routinely is in large part due to expense, lack of availability, and the research status of some of the tests. We suspect, however, that functional brain-imaging tests to assess concussion will be the way of the future.

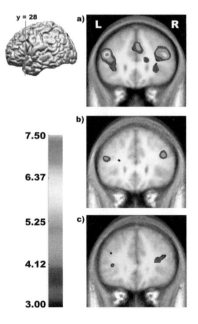

FIGURE 3.7   Average brain activation patterns during a verbal working memory task in *(a)* control subjects, *(b)* concussed athletes with mild postconcussive symptoms (PCS), and *(c)* concussed athletes with moderate PCS. Note the reduction in brain activity in the mild PCS group and even more pronounced reduction in the moderate PCS group.

Courtesy of Jen-Kai Chen, Alain Ptito PhD, and Karen Johnston MD, PhD.

Sport-related concussions usually do not cause gross structural damage (which is why the structural CT or MRI is usually normal), but they do typically cause functional (and usually reversible) impairment in brain cells. The physician evaluating a concussed athlete typically makes a decision about the necessity of a structural-imaging scan based on clinical signs and symptoms, along with the individual's medical and concussion history.

It is important to realize that a CT or MRI of the head is not always indicated (in medical and health insurance company terms, "not medically necessary") in the routine assessment of many sport concussions. Studies show that these structural-imaging studies are read as normal over 90% of the time after a mild sport concussion. Dr. Jeff Bazarian (2004), an associate professor of emergency medicine at the University of Rochester Medical Center, cited published studies that provide guidelines for determining the need for CT in the emergency department for children, adolescents, and adults with mild TBI (not restricted to sport concussion). For children and adolescents, a CT is warranted if any of these three signs and symptoms are present: change in mental status, vomiting, or signs of skull fracture. For adults with mild TBI, any of the following signs and symptoms warrant a CT scan of the head: persistent anterograde amnesia, drug or alcohol intoxication, age greater than 60 years, seizure or vomiting, and signs of trauma above the clavicles. These guidelines were reported to be 98% and 100% sensitive and specific for children and adolescents with mTBI, respectively, and 45% and 25% sensitive and specific in adults, respectively, for detecting abnormalities on a head CT.

In the United States, if an athlete or his parent insists on getting a CT or MRI of the brain, they *may* be responsible for the cost of it themselves. The most recent figures indicate that a routine CT scan of the head cost 1,500 dollars; and a head MRI was 3,000 dollars (not including the fees of the radiologist, who reads the CT and MRI results). And whether we like it or not, most high school and collegiate athletes do not get the quality and quantity of health care that professional athletes receive. Just because a prominent NFL running back tweaks a knee and is sent for an MRI doesn't mean that an MRI is the standard of medical care for *all* running backs who tweak a knee.

So, should someone insist on getting a head CT or MRI after a sport-related concussion? If you can afford it (or your insurance company will cover it), go ahead. Even if the scan is negative, it can be used as a structural baseline of the athlete's brain in case of future head trauma or brain disease. If the emergency department physician decides that a CT or MRI scan is unnecessary and an athlete is uncomfortable with the doctor's opinion, get a second opinion from a trusted family doctor or a specialized doctor experienced with concussion before incurring the expenses of these scans.

Neuropsychological Testing

Neuropsychological tests (also known as neurocognitive tests) are indirect measures of brain functioning via paper and pencil, question and answer, or computer-based tests. In sport concussion the tests measure memory, attention and concentration, learning, quickness of thinking and information processing, motor skills, and reaction time. This is just a partial list; neuropsychological tests measure other brain functions as well.

Neuropsychological tests were first utilized in clinical medicine in the 1940s. Bender and colleagues (2004) reported that the beginnings of neuropsychological testing for sport concussion, although not particularly clear, probably began in boxing. Dr. Jeff Barth and colleagues first used neuropsychological tests with collegiate athletes on a formal basis in the late 1980s. To our knowledge, the Pittsburgh Steelers were the first professional sports organization to use neuropsychological tests systematically in 1993. The Steelers' team neurosurgeon, Dr. Joseph Maroon, was instrumental in having neuropsychologist Dr. Mark Lovell adapt clinical neuropsychological tests for use with the Steelers for the assessment of concussion. Neuropsychological tests were first used in the NHL in 1997 as a research protocol, again under the direction and leadership of Dr. Lovell.

The utility and validity of neuropsychological testing for the assessment of sport-related concussion has been demonstrated in numerous published scientific studies (see the Research Digest section at the end of this chapter). Neuropsychological testing is being used currently by many sport organizations and professionals including the NHL, the NFL, several National Basketball Association and Major League Baseball teams, NCAA sports, Major League Baseball umpires, the Olympics, soccer, rugby, CART and IRL racing, NASCAR, and others. The list continues to grow. It should be noted, however, that some neuropsychologists question the utility of neuropsychological testing in sport-related concussion (Randolph et al. in press).

Neuropsychological testing in sports generally uses an individual baseline approach because athletes vary considerably in cognitive abilities. Athletes are tested prior to the beginning of the season, and retested after a concussion. The selected tests are sensitive to the effects of cerebral concussion and measure verbal and visual learning and memory, concentration, speed of information processing, and eye-hand coordination. Comparisons are made between baseline scores and postconcussion scores on an individualized basis. Test scores can be used to assess the severity of the concussion and to track recovery over time.

Various paper-and-pencil batteries have been constructed by neuropsychologists for baseline and postconcussion testing; these have been adapted from neuropsychological tests used in routine clinical practice. Two examples are listed in the Research Digest.

Computer-based platforms developed specifically for sport concussion are now available for baseline and postconcussion testing. Among these platforms is the Immediate Postconcussion Assessment and Cognitive Testing (ImPACT), developed by Drs. Mark Lovell, Joseph Maroon, and others at the University of Pittsburgh Medical Center. Dr. David Erlanger and colleagues in New York developed the Concussion Resolution Index (CRI, a part of Head-Minder). CRI is a popular, web-based computer program for the assessment of sport concussion. Dr. Alexander Collie and his associates in Australia developed CogSport (now known as Concussion Sentinel), another popular computer-based assessment tool. Web sites and addresses for these sport-concussion computer platforms are available in appendix B. See Podell (2004) for an excellent discussion of the use of computerized neuropsychological testing for sport concussion.

Neuropsychological tests are most useful when a preseason baseline has been obtained so that individualized comparisons can be made. The introduction of computer-based tests has made baseline neuropsychological testing available and affordable to most athletic organizations. McCrory (2004) reviewed the literature on the evidence base for recommendations regarding pre-athletic-participation assessment for head injury. McCrory reported that expert consensus indicated that a baseline neuropsychological evaluation, preferably with a computerized battery, was indicated.

We concur and strongly recommend baseline neuropsychological testing on all athletes at all levels of competition.

Are Neuropsychological Test Results Fallible?

Yes. These tests are imperfect measures of brain functioning. Keep in mind that no single test (or test battery) can capture all aspects of brain functioning. Test results can be affected adversely by anxiety, poor effort on testing, personality issues, or other environmental or situational factors (for example, testing an athlete in a noisy locker room). Neuropsychologists typically do not have time (or permission) to do baseline testing on all these factors and account for all possible variables, just as a physician cannot perform all possible medical tests on every player. There are also advantages and disadvantages to the type of neuropsychological tests used (for example, sideline screening measures versus paper-and-pencil tests versus computerized batteries), but a discussion of those issues may be relevant only to neuropsychologists. Such discussions are available in the professional neuropsychological literature for those who are interested.

Is the Neuropsychologist Fallible?

Absolutely. Just as the ATC, the physician, and the rest of us are fallible, the neuropsychologist may have varying levels of expertise in assessing the test results in sport concussion. Psychologists (in general) are bound by an ethical code that precludes them from providing services for which they may not have the appropriate training and experience (exceptions are made in emergency circumstances). The routine use of neuropsychological testing for the assessment of sport concussion is an endeavor that is just over a decade old. Given its relative newness, there may not be a large number of appropriately trained and experienced neuropsychologists available to provide these services. Do not hesitate to ask the neuropsychologist about her experience with sport concussion.

When the NHL's clinical research neuropsychological testing program was introduced in 1997 (see page 74), one aspect of the program was that each team's neuropsychologist consulted with a supervising neuropsychologist for review of the test data on every concussion. That component is still in effect, and it is quite helpful in ensuring that test results are interpreted as accurately as possible.

It is encouraging to see neuropsychologists seek collaborative consultation to ensure an athlete's safety postconcussion.

Role of Grading Scales in Assessment

The true values of a concussion-grading scale are in its ability to classify severity of concussion accurately and to offer useful prognostic information, including return-to-play criteria. Unfortunately, these goals have not been met consistently with most concussion-grading systems. Indeed, in 1999 Dr. Paul McCrory wrote an article in which he listed eleven myths of sport concussion, one of which was "The myth of concussion-grading scales" (p. 136). More than 25 concussion-grading scales are available in the medical literature. For a review of these scales, see the article by Dr. Karen Johnston and colleagues (2001b) in the *Clinical Journal of Sport Medicine*. Only Dr. Robert Cantu's Evidence-Based Rating Scale (2001) has been reported as based on empirical study. All other scales have been based on clinical experience and expert consensus opinion (which are valuable, but viewed as less compelling in scientific circles).

The most frequently used grading scales in the past have included those of Dr. Cantu (1986, 2001) and the 1997 American Academy of Neurology (AAN) Practice Parameter (which was an expansion of the 1991 Colorado Medical Society Guidelines). There are advantages and disadvantages to each scale. Let's take a look a little more in depth at these commonly used scales.

Cantu's Concussion-Grading Scales

Dr. Robert Cantu published his first grading scale in 1986, and he presented his revised, evidence-based rating scale in a 2001 issue of the *Journal of Athletic Training*. A mild, or Grade 1, concussion involves no loss of consciousness (LOC) and posttraumatic amnesia (defined as either anterograde or retrograde amnesia) or postconcussion signs and symptoms lasting less than 30 minutes. A Grade 2, or moderate, concussion involves LOC of less than 1 minute and posttraumatic amnesia or postconcussion signs and symptoms lasting longer than 30 minutes but less than 24 hours. A Grade 3, or severe, concussion involves LOC lasting more than 1 minute or posttraumatic amnesia lasting longer than 24 hours, along with postconcussion signs and symptoms lasting longer than 7 days. Dr. Cantu hastens to add that a concussion cannot be graded accurately with his evidence-based scale until all symptoms have cleared.

Grading Scale of the American Academy of Neurology

The American Academy of Neurology (AAN; 1997) defined a Grade 1 concussion as involving transient confusion, no LOC, and resolution of concussion symptoms or mental status abnormalities within 15 minutes. A Grade 2 concussion was defined as transient confusion, no LOC, and concussion symptoms or mental status abnormalities lasting more than 15 minutes. A Grade 3 concussion was defined as involving any LOC, be it either brief (seconds) or prolonged (minutes).

Return-to-Play Recommendations

Most of the popular grading systems for concussion also contain return-to-play (RTP) recommendations. After all, the true value of a grading system is in its ability to categorize concussion severity accurately *and* to provide useful clinical management strategies (like RTP criteria). And the RTP recommendations for each system tend to be tied to the concussion grade. For example, in a Grade 1 concussion (and assuming it to be an athlete's first of the season), Cantu recommends RTP if the athlete has no symptoms for a week. The AAN system recommends RTP within the same contest if the player's symptoms or mental status abnormalities clear within 15 minutes. However, a second Grade 1 concussion within the same contest eliminates the player from competition that day (according to AAN), with RTP based on the player being symptom free for one week.

For a Grade 2 concussion, AAN recommends that an athlete should not return to play until he or she has been symptom free for at least two weeks, both at rest and after exertion. Cantu recommends that following a Grade 2 concussion, an athlete may return to play after one week if the athlete is asymptomatic, at rest and after exertion. However, if this is the athlete's second concussion of the season (irrespective of grade), Cantu recommends withholding the athlete from competition for one month, with return to play allowed if the athlete is symptom free for another week. If this is the athlete's third concussion in a season, Cantu recommends terminating the season for that athlete with return to play during the next season if the athlete is asymptomatic.

For a Grade 3 concussion, AAN guidelines restrict a player from RTP for one week if LOC was brief (seconds) and for two weeks if LOC was prolonged (minutes). Cantu's system recommends no RTP for a minimum of one month with a Grade 3 concussion.

A recent study by Dr. Mark Lovell and associates (2004) muddies the waters even further when dealing with Grade 1 concussions and RTP issues. Recall that the AAN guidelines allow for RTP in the same game if an athlete sustains a first (in that season) concussion and the symptoms clear within 15 minutes. Lovell studied 43 high school athletes who sustained a Grade 1 concussion and had resolution of symptoms within 15 minutes (but were not allowed to RTP during that contest). All athletes had undergone preseason baseline neuropsychological testing and a symptom checklist. All athletes were readministered the neuropsychological tests and symptom checklist twice during the week following the concussion. Results indicated that 36 hours postconcussion the concussed athletes demonstrated a decline on memory testing and a dramatic increase in self-reported symptoms when compared with baseline data. Athletes "demonstrated memory deficits and symptoms that persisted beyond the context in which they were injured." Lovell and colleagues note that "these data suggest that current grade 1 return-to-play recommendations that allow for immediate return to play may be too liberal" (p. 47).

It gets more complicated when it is the athlete's second or third concussion in a season, and even more confusing when the athlete's concussions are not all the same grade. For example, does a Grade 1 concussion plus a Grade 2 concussion sustained 2 weeks later add up to more than a single Grade 3 concussion? Do three separate Grade 1 concussions in a season equal one Grade 3 concussion? Are multiple concussions additive or exponential?

The essential point to be made here is that RTP recommendations are generally tied to the concussion-grading system utilized, and not all grading systems are the same. So a Grade 1 concussion for an athlete on one team may not be the same as a Grade 1 concussion for an athlete on a different team. Similarly, the RTP expectations for an athlete on team A may be different from the RTP expectations for an athlete on team B. It depends, of course, on which grading system (and RTP recommendations) the sports medicine professional utilizes. We also believe that an athlete's age may be a relevant factor, with more conservative management needed for younger athletes. But given that the majority of published grading systems have traditionally weighed LOC too heavily, we now know the systems are probably misleading.

Compounding the issue further was a study by Dr. Melvin Field and colleagues (2003), published in the *Journal of Pediatrics*. Baseline neuropsychological testing and symptom checklists were completed on high school and collegiate athletes. Approximately 10% of each group sustained concussions. The authors found that the concussed high school athletes performed worse on the memory tests than the collegiate athletes, pointing toward the variable of age as an important determinant of recovery from concussion.

Regarding the prognostic value of concussion-grading scales, an initial study by Drs. Hinton-Bayre and Geffen (2002), published in the *British Journal of Sports Medicine,* is quite relevant. These authors obtained baseline neuropsychological test data on professional athletes and matched controls. Each concussed player was assigned a concussion severity grade based on three different published concussion-grading scales. Results indicated that concussion severity, as assessed by the various guidelines, was not related to subsequent neuropsychological outcome. The authors concluded that current classifications of concussion severity did not predict short-term neuropsychological status.

Concussion grading scales are one area in which the multidisciplinary aspect of sports medicine becomes a double-edged sword. Although we've seen no studies on the topic, we have to wonder what goes in to the decision made by a sports medicine professional about which grading system to use. It would seem that in the spirit of professional identification (and possibly medicolegal concerns), neurologists will utilize the AAN parameters, and neurosurgeons are more likely to follow Cantu's guidelines (Cantu is a neurosurgeon). Will neuropsychologists and ATCs invent their own scales? Or as McCrory (1999) commented, "Doctors, coaches, and athletes can 'shop around' for an injury scale and advice about returning to play that suits their sporting needs but which may not be the best medical management for their injury" (p. 136).

We don't know the answers to these questions, and we're not sure that anyone else does either. Each concussion must be evaluated and treated individually. This need for an individualized approach is why the Concussion in Sport Group (CIS 2002) did not recommend the use of any particular grading system and set out RTP criteria that were essentially separate from any grading of concussion (explained in chapter 4, page 63).

How Long Does It Take to Recover From a Concussion?

Ideally, the expected rate of recovery postconcussion is what a truly accurate grading scale would tell us. Unfortunately, there is no simple answer to this question because not all concussions are the same. A recent prospective study of collegiate football players ("The NCAA Concussion Study"; McCrea et al. 2003) sheds some light on this question. Concussed players experienced more symptoms, cognitive impairment, and balance problems than control players immediately after a concussion. On average, the balance deficits remitted by days 3 to 5, cognitive functioning returned to baseline by days 5 to 7, and subjective symptoms gradually resolved by day 7. The mild neuropsychological impairments in verbal memory and cognitive processing noted on day 2 resolved by day 7. No group differences were noted on any of the outcome measures by day 90. In essence, the NCAA study suggests that most football concussions resolve within a week.

Pellman and associates (2004a), in their article on concussion in NFL players (to be discussed in greater detail in chapter 5), reported that the majority of those concussions cleared within 6 days. And, in a prospective study of 729 athletes who sustained a boxing concussion, Dr. Joseph Bleiberg and colleagues (2004) reported that cognitive recovery typically occurred by 3 to 7 days postinjury.

In an article in *Current Sports Medicine Reports*, Cantu (2003) offered "absolute" and "relative" contraindications for a return to collision practice or competition (in other words, RTP). Absolute contraindications included any of the following:

- Abnormal findings on neurological examination
- Presence of postconcussion symptoms at rest or with exertion

- "Below-baseline" neuropsychological test results
- CT or MRI showing a lesion

Relative contraindications for RTP included the following:

- Duration of postconcussion symptoms lasting for months
- Mild, indirect blow (whiplash type injury not directly to the head) producing significant postconcussion symptoms

The variability in concussion recovery rates is astounding. Some athletes have their symptoms clear within minutes, whereas others have waited a year or more for their symptoms to dissipate. On the *average*, recovery probably takes about 7 days. This figure will be affected by a multitude of variables, including age, prior concussion history, concurrent medical problems, and other factors. Again, each concussion must be considered individually.

Research Digest

For an overview of the McGill protocol, see the article by Drs. Johnston, Lassonde, and Ptito in a 2000 issue of the *Journal of the American College of Surgeons.*

The Sport Concussion Assessment Tool (SCAT) was derived from the following: the Sideline Evaluation for Concussion of the Colorado Head Injury Foundation, the Standardized Assessment of Concussion (McCrea et al. 1997), the Management of Concussion in Sports Palm Card of the American Academy of Neurology and the Brain Injury Association, the Sideline Concussion Check of the UPMC Sport Concussion Program, ThinkSafe and Sports Medicine New Zealand and the Brain Injury Association, the McGill Abbreviated Concussion Evaluation (ACE), and the National Hockey League Physician Evaluation Form.

Clinicians who use balance testing (the BESS in particular) would benefit from reviewing a study done by Dr. Tamara Valovich and associates, which was published in a 2003 issue of the *Journal of Athletic Training,* and a separate study done by Joseph Wilkins, ATC, and associates (2004). Valovich found a learning, or practice, effect (improved performance on a test simply as a function of repeated exposure to the test) on the BESS in healthy high school athletes. Wilkins found that fatigue alone could account for decreased performance on the BESS and recommended that clinicians using the BESS as part of their sideline assessment for concussion should not administer the BESS immediately after a concussion due to the effects of fatigue.

For a review of the role of structural neuroimaging in sport concussion, see the article by Johnston and associates in the *Clinical Journal of Sport Medicine* (2001c). Scientific studies attesting to the validity and utility of neuropsychological testing in the assessment of sport-related concussion can be found in Collie et al. (2003), Collins and associates (1999), Echemendia et al. (2001), Grindell and associates (2001), Lovell (2002), and Lovell and Collins (1998).

The neuropsychological test battery for the NHL initially utilized the Post-Concussion Scale-Revised (PCS-R), Orientation Test, Hopkins Verbal Learning Test-Revised (Hopkins), Ruff Figural Fluency Test, Controlled Oral Word Association Test (COWAT), Symbol Digit Modalities, Penn State Cancellation Test, and Color Trails Test. The Ruff was replaced with the Brief Visuospatial Memory Test-Revised (BVMT-R) in 2000. The initial NFL neuropsychological test battery utilized the PCS-R, Orientation Test, the Digit Span, Digit Symbol, and Symbol Search subtests from the Wechsler Adult Intelligence Scale-III, COWAT, Hopkins, and BVMT-R.

In the Field et al. (2003) study, there were 371 collegiate athletes (mean age 19.9 years) and 183 high school athletes (mean age 15.9 years). Thirty-five of the collegiate (9.4%) and 19 (10.4%) of the high school athletes sustained a concussion. The majority of the concussions were classified as Grade 1 or Grade 2 according to American Academy of Neurology (AAN) criteria.

In the Hinton-Bayre and Geffen (2002) study, there were 21 professional rugby players and 21 matched controls. Concussion-severity grades were based on the Cantu (1986), Colorado Medical Society (1990), and AAN (1997) guidelines.

The two NCAA concussion studies (Guskiewicz et al. 2003; McCrea et al. 2003) involved 1,631 football players from 15 U.S. colleges (including Divisions I, II, and III) over 3 football seasons (1999 to 2001). All players underwent preseason baseline testing with a concussion-symptom checklist, the Standardized Assessment of Concussion (SAC), the Balance Error Scoring System

(BESS), and selected neuropsychological tests. Of the 94 athletes (5.76%) who sustained a concussion, 79 (84%) completed the protocol. Controls for the study comprised 56 uninjured athletes. All players (injured and control subjects) completed the tests immediately; 3 hours; and 1, 2, 3, 5, 7, and 90 days after injury.

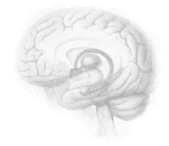

chapter 4

Treatment and Rehabilitation

In this chapter we discuss medical and nonmedical treatments for concussion and address the issue of what can be done about concussion. We also look at the interrelationships between concussion symptoms and the results of neuroimaging and neuropsychological testing.

Medical Treatments for Concussion

In the United States there is no medical treatment for concussion that has been approved by the Food and Drug Administration (FDA). Dr. Paul McCrory (2001c) concluded the following in a summary article on this topic in the *Clinical Journal of Sport Medicine*: "At the present time, the clinician has no evidence-based pharmacological treatment to offer the concussed athlete" (p. 190). Dr. McCrory's conclusion is similar to that made by the American Orthopedic Society for Sports Medicine in 1999 (Wojtys et al.). The workshop participants concluded, "At the current time, there are no curative treatments for concussion and the best approach to management of concussion emphasizes early recognition of postconcussive symptoms and prevention of additional concussive injury"

(p. 681). Interestingly, however, in the series of articles on concussion in the National Football League (NFL), 1.4% of concussed athletes received "prescription drug therapy," and 0.6% received a "proprietary prescription" (Pellman et al. 2004b). No mention was made of the specific drugs used.

The overwhelming majority of clinical pharmacological efforts at treating concussion have been for people with severe brain injuries. Other studies have utilized animal models of human head trauma. Dr. McCrory (2001c) grouped findings (based on all available human data) into three categories. The first was those drugs viewed as "possibly effective" (at some point in the future). These included corticosteroids (for example, methylprednisolone), calcium channel antagonists, opiate receptor antagonists, and drugs inhibiting arachidonic acid metabolism. The second category was those drugs viewed as "unlikely to be effective," which included neurotrophic factors (such as growth hormone) and thyrotropin-releasing hormone. A third category was "treatments that may place the athlete at risk of adverse events." Drugs in this category included free-radical scavengers and antioxidants (for example, vitamins E and C), drugs that modify monoamine function (compounds that act on a group of naturally occurring brain enzymes), and glutamate-receptor antagonists (chemicals that block the release of glutamate in the brain after a concussion). Dr. McCrory also addressed the possible uses of hypothermia and hyperbaric-oxygen therapy in his review of possible treatments for concussion. At the time he discussed his findings (2001c), neither treatment could be recommended by McCrory for the treatment of concussion.

In the United States, the FDA approves drugs for specific medical conditions. Any use of the drug for purposes other than the approved medical conditions is referred to as "off-label" uses. Physicians vary considerably in their practices with the off-label use of drugs. Over the years we have read case studies or heard anecdotal reports of many drugs being used (with varying degrees of success) in the off-label treatment of head injury (not necessarily sport-related concussion). See the Research Digest section for a list of some of these drugs. *Note:* Always consult an informed physician about any treatment for concussion. The potential risks and benefits of any drug treatment should be explored thoroughly before beginning treatment.

Nonmedical Management and Rehabilitation

The Concussion in Sport (CIS) Group (2002, 2005) developed recommendations for the treatment of concussion, which have essentially gleaned the successful elements common to various rehabilitative protocols in their approach. The CIS group agreed that a structured and supervised rehabilitative protocol would be conducive to optimal recovery and safe and successful return to play. Instead of endorsing a specific protocol, CIS focused on common principles found in various rehabilitative programs. They recommended that the athlete be completely free of symptoms and have normal neurological and cognitive evaluations prior to the start of a rehabilitative program. A stepwise progression with gradual, incremental increases in exercise intensity and duration was recommended, along with a backtracking (or stepping down) with any recurrence of symptoms. It was estimated that each step in the process might take a minimum of one day. However, proceeding successfully through the steps will be dependent on the individual athlete. Here are the steps recommended by CIS:

Step 1: No activity with complete rest until all symptoms resolve

Step 2: Light aerobic exercises such as walking or stationary cycling

Step 3: Sport-specific training, such as running in soccer or skating in hockey

Step 4: Noncontact training drills

Step 5: After medical clearance, full contact training

Step 6: Game play

CIS recommended that if an athlete completes a step without the recurrence of concussion symptoms, then he should proceed to the next level. If the athlete experiences any recurrence of concussion symptoms, the athlete should drop back to the prior step and try to progress again after 24 hours. It is important to note that symptoms may not recur during exercise but may be worse later, or especially the next day. Rehabilitation programs need to be tailored to the individual athlete and her symptoms. The ATC, in conjunction with a medical doctor experienced in the treatment of concussion, is probably best qualified to construct a rehabilitation program for the concussed athlete.

The primary nonmedical treatment for concussion is rest and the avoidance of exertion (both physical *and* mental) until the symptoms have resolved completely. The primary purpose of rest is to allow the brain to recover fully and to prevent the occurrence of another concussion before the brain has healed. Most sports medicine clinicians are aware that exertional *physical* activity can provoke symptoms of concussion. Many are less aware, however, that exertional *cognitive* activity can do the same. Neuropsychologists who perform cognitive assessments on concussed athletes are all too familiar with athletes developing headaches or other concussion-related symptoms during (or immediately after) taking the cognitive tests. It is important to minimize exertional cognitive activities in symptomatic concussed athletes during the acute recovery phase. High school and collegiate athletes may need to be excused from academic classes or afforded accommodations (for example, more time to complete an assignment, tape recording of lectures).

If baseline neuropsychological testing has been done, we expect the athlete's scores to have returned to baseline before beginning any physical rehabilitation. Once all symptoms have resolved at rest, and the neuropsychological test scores have returned to baseline, an athlete may then begin a step-by-step rehabilitative program of graduated, increased activity under the supervision of a trainer or physician until he or she returns to game-ready condition.

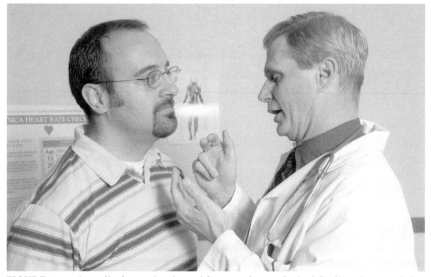

FIGURE 4.1   A medical examination with normal neurological findings is essential before an athlete returns to play.

The recommendation of rest typically doesn't go over very well with athletes, who are trained to be active and conditioned to play hurt. Athletes feel nearly compelled to exercise strained muscles; unfortunately, as Dr. Mark Lovell has said, the brain is not a muscle. Nonetheless, these guidelines were the recommendation of the CIS group and have become the standard of care for most sports medicine professionals working with sport concussion. Athletes typically learn (the hard way) that if they attempt a return to play before complete resolution of all symptoms at rest and on exertion, the symptoms often recur and frequently with greater intensity. In our opinion and experience, the complete resolution of symptoms actually takes longer if an athlete returns to play prematurely and experiences a temporary worsening of symptoms. And, in general, the longer the symptoms persist, the longer the periods of rest and rehabilitation will be required.

We have also found it useful (in consultation with the trainer and team physician) to make several other recommendations to athletes during their rehabilitation from concussion. First, because athletes are not particularly good at sitting still and doing nothing, we frequently recommend that they try activities that focus on breathing, toning, and stretching. Many athletes have worked with sport psychologists in the past and have learned some form of relaxation or visualization technique. We encourage athletes to practice these skills but emphasize that they should omit the tensing and relaxing of muscle groups (which is a part of some relaxation techniques) to avoid exerting themselves. The exertion in this type of relaxation strategy can worsen the symptoms of concussion. It is also important to delay resistance training and weightlifting until later in the rehabilitation protocol. It has been noted frequently that postconcussion symptoms readily recur with weightlifting, even though it is not aerobic and athletes don't always think of it as exertion.

A report by Bloom and colleagues suggests advantages to sport psychology interventions in concussion (2004). This is a new area of research, but the potential benefits offer an exciting new approach to the management of concussion. Also, sport-specific concussion rehabilitation protocols, described as "multidimensional concussion rehabilitation," are being developed in an effort to optimize each player's technique and skill while recovering from concussive injury (Johnston et al. 2004).

Management of specific common symptoms is also warranted. For example, we suggest the routine use of sunglasses if it is bright outside, particularly for those athletes whose concussion symptoms include headache or sensitivity to light (photophobia). For athletes with photophobia we have used a graduated exposure approach using light boxes typically utilized for people with seasonal depression. We also recommend that athletes avoid extremely noisy places, especially if sensitivity to noise (phonophobia) is a symptom of concern. An alternative is to wear earplugs in noisy places. In addition, we caution athletes about the use of alcohol, as many individuals are more sensitive to the effects of alcohol after a concussion. Over-the-counter analgesics (for example, acetaminophen, ibuprofen) should be used prudently and in consultation with a physician. Finally, we do some basic counseling and education about concussion with the athlete (and family, if available). Our approach is to emphasize the fact that 90% of the time, concussion is a self-limiting phenomenon that runs its course and concludes with a complete recovery.

Comparing Symptoms and Assessment Results

The scientific evaluation, assessment, and treatment of concussion are far from fully explored. We are just beginning to disentangle and understand the myriad factors associated with this often confusing area of sports medicine. It is not uncommon for even seasoned sports medicine professionals to have questions about the multiple factors and features of a concussion. Given that treatment and rehabilitation often depend on the outcomes of concussion-assessment strategies, it may be helpful to take a look at some of the more common questions we have received over the years from athletes, trainers, physicians, and sports-management personnel:

• **How often do the neuropsychological test results and the player's symptoms agree?** Generally speaking, according to the experience at the University of Pittsburgh's Sports Concussion Program, the results are concordant approximately 75% of the time.

• **Why don't the neuropsychological test results and the player's symptoms agree 100% of the time?** Several explanations are possible. First, many athletes underreport their symptoms. They want to play, and their mentality is one of playing hurt. They know that another player is waiting to fill their shoes if they cannot play. It is not uncommon for an athlete to deny the presence of any postconcussion symptoms whatsoever and then do extremely poorly on the neuropsychological tests. In this case, the neuropsychological tests may catch or identify an athlete who is underreporting symptoms and is still suffering from a concussive injury.

Neuropsychological tests do not have perfect sensitivity, however, and it is not uncommon that those test scores may have returned to baseline while symptoms persist. This finding is one reason why formal assessment of postconcussion symptoms is so essential. In rare cases, athletes may overreport symptoms (for a variety of psychological reasons). These factors may also lead to a lack of agreement between symptoms and test scores.

- **How can a player still have symptoms yet have a normal MRI?** The MRI measures structure of the brain, not function. Stretching and tearing of axons (a part of the neuron) usually do not show up on a structural MRI (individual neurons are too small to be seen with the naked eye or with MRI). Over 100,000 axons can fit easily on half of a fingernail. Microscopic analysis would be required to view any possible pathological changes in the cells. Just because the MRI is normal does not always mean that everything is fine; it means that certain pathological conditions have been ruled out.

- **How can the MRI be normal and the neuropsychological tests be abnormal?** Neuropsychological tests are sensitive to both functional and structural damage to nerve cells. The MRI may show no structural damage to nerve cells, but the neuropsychological tests can detect the functional impairments of the cells most of the time.

- **How can the MRI and neuropsychological tests be normal and the player still have symptoms?** There are multiple possibilities here. One is that the structural MRI and the neuropsychological tests are not sensitive enough to pick up some subtle functional impairment in the nerve cells. In this case we have seen that the *fMRI* can be abnormal. Current research indicates that when the clinical symptoms cease, the fMRI abnormalities remit.

A second possibility has to do with "practice effects" on the paper-and-pencil neuropsychological tests. Repeated exposure to these tests often results in improved performance simply from taking them so frequently (the practice effect). So an athlete's neuropsychological test scores may be at baseline when the athlete's brain isn't. The new computer-based neuropsychological tests limit this problem of practice effects.

A third (and more remote) possibility is that a player is magnifying or exaggerating symptoms, possibly for psychological reasons (for example, the person wants time off, fears another hit, or is dealing with other psychological issues). In our experience, this is the exception, not the rule.

Research Digest

Here is a partial list of drugs (with examples) used in the off-label treatment of head injury (not necessarily sport-related concussion):

Tricyclic antidepressants (TCAs): nortriptyline, amitriptyline

Psychostimulants: methylphenidate

Serotonin selective reuptake inhibitors (SSRIs): sertraline, fluoxetine, paroxetine

Serotonin-norepinephrine selective reuptake inhibitors (SNRIs): venlafaxine, duloxetine

Dopamine agonists: amantadine

Acetylcholinesterase inhibitors (AchIs): donepezil, galantamine, rivastigmine

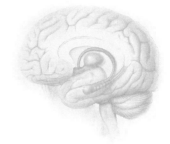

chapter 5

Concussion in Professional Sports

In this chapter we discuss sport-specific concussion. Summary information from the National Football League (NFL) and the National Hockey League (NHL) is presented as well as overviews from the sports of soccer and boxing. We address data on concussion from professional and nonprofessional athletes in the sections on soccer and boxing. A section on heading the ball in soccer is included, given that this topic has been an area of heated debate.

Concussion in the National Football League

Dr. Joseph Maroon, the team neurosurgeon for the Pittsburgh Steelers, is fond of telling a story of how neuropsychological testing began in the NFL. In the early 1990s, the Steelers' quarterback sustained a concussion. Dr. Maroon recommended that the athlete sit out for a week prior to returning to play. Chuck Knoll, head coach of the Steelers, asked Dr. Maroon about the scientific basis of his recommendation. According to Knoll's perception, his quarterback had recovered fully, was showing no postconcussion signs or symptoms, and thus was able to play. Dr. Maroon replied that his recommendation was based on the prevailing neurosurgical standard of care at that time. When Coach Knoll asked for the scientific basis of the prevailing standard of care, Dr. Maroon was at a loss to provide any data other than expert opinion. Dr. Maroon then contacted neuropsychologist Dr. Mark Lovell, and shortly thereafter the Steelers began conducting baseline neuropsychological testing. Interestingly, the impetus for the use of neuropsychological testing in the NFL came from a head coach.

In 1994 Paul Tagliabue, the commissioner of the NFL, formed a committee to study scientifically the issue of concussion in its players. The NFL Committee on Mild Traumatic Brain Injuries comprised representatives from the NFL Team Physicians Society; the NFL Athletic Trainers Society; NFL equipment managers; and external scientific consultants in the specialty areas of **neuropsychology**, **epidemiology**, neurology, neurosurgery, and biomechanical engineering. Between 1996 and 2001, nearly 900 cases were compiled with detailed assessments of the impact, players, equipment worn, follow-up medical treatments, and return-to-play data. Commissioner Tagliabue published an overview of this process in the journal *Neurosurgery* (2003).

The first of the published studies resulting from the 5-year project was titled "Concussion in Professional Football: Reconstruction of Game Impacts and Injuries" and appeared in the October 2003 issue of *Neurosurgery* by Dr. Elliot Pellman and colleagues. Dr. Pellman served as chair of the NFL Committee on Mild Traumatic Brain Injuries. The first paper was dedicated to an explanation of the data collection and laboratory reconstruction methods used in the study.

The second paper ("Concussion in Professional Football: Location and Direction of Helmet Impacts") appeared in the December 2003 issue of *Neurosurgery*. The article reports in detail the results of exhaustive analyses of 182 NFL concussions, with laboratory reconstruction of 31 impacts via helmeted hybrid dummies (similar to the types used in automobile crash tests). The results showed that 71% of the impacts are to the side of the helmet shell primarily from another player's helmet (see figure 5.1), arm, or shoulder or from ground contact to the back of the head. The remainder of the impacts (29%) was primarily from helmet contact to the face mask at an oblique frontal angle. These data

neuropsychology—A branch of psychology that is devoted to the scientific study of brain-behavior relationships.

epidemiology—The study of the relationships of the various factors determining the frequency and distribution of disease or injury in a human community.

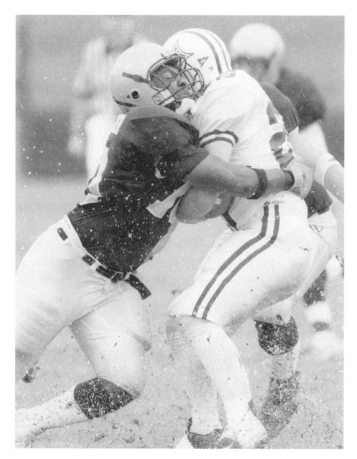

FIGURE 5.1 Head-to-head impact in football.
Photo courtesy of Mark Cohen.

indicate that spearing (a football tackling practice in which the crown of the helmet is used as a weapon and as the initial point of contact) has not been eliminated from football after all; and, according to these studies, spearing is the leading cause of concussion in the NFL.

Laboratory reconstruction revealed that concussions in the NFL occurred with a **G-force** of 78 to 117. The most common signs and symptoms experienced by concussed players were headaches, dizziness, immediate recall (memory) problems, and difficulty with information processing.

The third article (Pellman et al. 2004a) reported on the epidemiological aspects of 787 game-related cases of

> **G-force (g)**—A physical measure of gravitational force.

concussion during the 1996 to 2001 seasons. Thirty of the 32 NFL teams participated in the study. The range of concussions per team over the study period was 6 to 72, with the median number being 26. The NFL averaged 0.41 reported concussions per game during this time period. We suspect the number of actual concussions per game may be higher.

The relative risk of concussion was highest for quarterbacks, followed by wide receivers, tight ends, and defensive backs. Impact by another player's helmet accounted for 67.7% of the concussions, and 20.9% occurred as a result of impact from other body regions of the striking player. The remaining 11.4% of concussions were due to ground contact.

The specific type of play was also relevant for the occurrence of concussion. The highest risk of sustaining a concussion was (in descending order) on kickoffs, punt returns, rushing plays, and passing plays. Players on special teams are thus at highest risk for concussions in the NFL.

In terms of reported clinical symptoms, the three most common were headaches, dizziness, and blurred vision. The three most common signs noted during physical examination by a physician were problems with immediate recall, retrograde amnesia (inability to remember events that occurred prior to the impact), and information-processing problems. In 58 of the 787 cases (9.3%), the player lost consciousness. (The 9% figure is virtually identical to the incidence of concussion with loss of consciousness [LOC] reported in high school and collegiate athletes by Guskiewicz and colleagues [2000]). Nineteen (2.4%) of the players in the Pellman study were hospitalized. One player had a seizure.

In terms of return-to-play outcomes, 346 players (44%) were removed from play, 127 (16.1%) returned to play immediately, and 280 (35.6%) rested and then returned to play. This next figure is noteworthy—51.7% of concussed NFL players returned to play in the same game. Over 90% of the concussed athletes returned to play in less than 6 days. Players experiencing LOC were held out of play 2.6 times longer than those whose concussion did not involve LOC.

The fourth article (Pellman et al. 2004b) focused on repeat concussions. About one fourth of the concussed players experienced a repeat injury during the 1996 to 2001 study period. About 8% incurred three or more concussions. The average time lag between concussions was about 1 year. Only six concussions occurred within 2 weeks of the index injury. Repeat concussions were more prevalent among defensive backs, the kicking units, and wide receivers. Ball return carriers on special teams and quarterbacks were the most likely to sustain repeat concussions. More than 90% of the athletes were treated clinically with rest, and 57.5% of those with second concussions returned to play within a day.

The fifth article by the Pellman group (2004c) addressed the 72 concussions (8.1% of the total) leading to 7 or more days of missed playing time. By position, the highest frequency occurred in quarterbacks, the return unit on special teams, and defensive secondary players. The signs and symptoms most common in this group of concussed athletes were disorientation to time, retrograde amnesia, fatigue, and cognitive problems. LOC occurred in 7.9% of these cases.

According to Pellman and colleagues (2003a), the "typical" NFL concussion occurs at 20.8 miles per hour with peak head acceleration of 98 g's. These numbers translate to about 14 kilowatts of electricity or about 18 horsepower. Naunheim and associates (2000) estimate the G-force in hockey to be 35. However, according to Guy Genin, professor of mechanical engineering at Washington University in St. Louis, the 35 g figure may be a serious underestimation. Dr. Genin (2004) notes that the G-force estimate of Naunheim and colleagues just cited was based on a nonchecking condition (meaning that a hockey player is not allowed to keep an opponent in check by physical means) in a high school athlete. Genin estimates that the G-force in a severe, head-to-head collision among professional hockey players could reach up to four times the G-force reported by Naunheim, or approximately 140 g. Keep in mind that the type of helmets worn by athletes in football and hockey differ significantly, with lesser head protection in hockey helmets. Also, hockey players may skate at speeds of up to 30 mph, which amounts to a potentially greater force than in football, where players travel at about 21 mph (Pellman et al. 2003a).

It is laudable that the NFL has committed time and resources to the systematic and scientific study of concussion in its athletes. We hope these scientific efforts continue. In particular, we would like to see NFL officials share the results of these studies with the NFL referees, in hopes of enforcing the rules against spearing more effectively and with greater regularity.

The National Athletic Trainers' Association published a position statement titled "Head-Down Contact and Spearing in Tackle Football" (Heck et al. 2004). Although this statement was made with the intention of decreasing the risk of cervical spine fractures and dislocations in particular, educating (and reeducating) football players about proper tackling technique could prevent some concussive injuries as well. A formal educational program designed to inform NFL athletes about the signs and symptoms of concussion also would be of value. Continuation of the work at the Center for the Study of Professional Athletes at the University of North Carolina at Chapel Hill will undoubtedly help us better understand the possible long-term consequences of concussion for professional football players.

Concussion in the National Hockey League

In 1997 an agreement was made by the National Hockey League (NHL) and the NHL Players' Association (NHLPA) to embark on a 5-year clinical research project titled "The National Hockey League Neuropsychological Testing Program." The program was an attempt to study concussion scientifically and individually among NHL players. Dr. Mark Lovell and Dr. Ruben Echemendia headed the neuropsychological testing portion of the project (see Lovell, Echemendia, and Burke 2004).

Each NHL player was administered a preseason (baseline) series of neuropsychological tests designed to assess the brain functions most susceptible to the effects of concussion (for example, attention and concentration, memory, and speed of information processing). A structured symptom checklist (the postconcussion scale) also was administered. Players rated the presence or absence of each symptom on a 0 to 6 scale of severity. A thorough concussion history also was obtained, along with other basic demographic data. Because athletes vary considerably in cognitive abilities, it was deemed essential to have an individualized baseline of each player's cognitive (neuropsychological) functioning and clinical symptoms.

Two basic neuropsychological test batteries were constructed: one for English-speaking players, and a second for those players whose primary language was not English. The baseline test battery took about 30 minutes to complete. A leaguewide network of neuropsychologists was established, with (at least) one serving each team. Players who experienced a concussion underwent repeat neuropsychological testing (with alternate test forms as appropriate) 24 to 48 hours, 5 days, and 7 days postinjury. The symptom checklist also was repeated at each testing. The course of symptoms and test scores was assessed for each concussed player, allowing for the objective assessment of subjective symptoms and neuropsychological test scores throughout the recovery period. This general neuropsychological testing approach is now a mandatory clinical service in the NHL.

Although the NHL clinical research project has been completed, the results are still pending. When the results become available, the wealth of data in this project will be extremely informative regarding the process of recovery from sport-related concussion in elite athletes.

Dr. Charles Burke, director of the NHL Concussion Program, reported at the 2002 Sport Concussion Conference in Pittsburgh on the mechanisms of concussive injury in the NHL. Contact with the boards, glass, and ice accounted for 42% of the concussions; an elbow or forearm to the head caused 21%; a shoulder to head contact led to 19%; fights caused 12%; and a puck or stick to the head led to 6%. If you examine the game situation in figure 5.2 closely, you can identify many of these mechanisms. Many sports

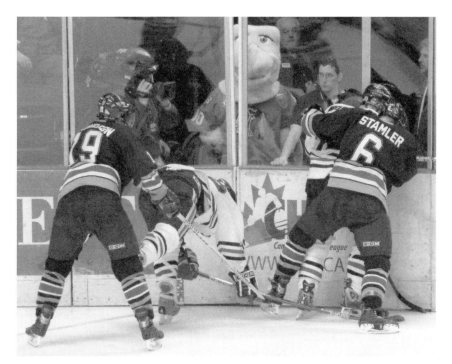

FIGURE 5.2　A typical situation during a hockey game.

medicine professionals thought that the seamless boards were a contributing factor to the increased number of concussions because these boards were too rigid on impact. These seamless boards were replaced in all NHL rinks by the start of the 2003-2004 season.

Wennberg and Tator (2003) compiled NHL concussion data from the years 1986 to 2002 using injury report data compiled by *The Hockey News.* Although collecting scientific data via media injury reporting has major obvious problems (such as difficulty discerning the true numbers), these numbers may reflect increased awareness of the injury, as pointed out by Johnston (2003) in an editorial in the *Canadian Journal of Neurological Sciences.* Between 1986 and 1996, there were anywhere from 7 to 17 concussions reported per season, leading to a NHL concussion rate ranging from 4 to 8 per 1,000 games. Since 1997 (the implementation date of the NHL Neuropsychological Testing Program), the number of reported concussions increased from 27 to 74 per season, leading to a concussion rate of 13 to 30 per 1,000 games. All statistics were adjusted for number of teams and games played per season. The authors report that the increased number of reported concussions was due, at least in part, to the greater awareness of the signs and symptoms of concussion brought about by the program.

At the 2004 Sport Concussion Conference in Pittsburgh, Dr. Burke reported that the annual number of NHL concussions for the years 1997 to 2003 ranged from 71 to 128 per year. The NHL Injury Analysis Committee performed a detailed video analysis on anywhere from 43 to 81 concussions per season. The number of concussions in the NHL is showing a downward trend.

We applaud the NHL and the NHLPA for their scientific and programmatic efforts to address the problem of concussion for its athletes. The NHLPA has taken a particularly proactive approach in educating its athletes about concussion. The proposal by Dr. Tom Pashby and colleagues (2001) calling for putting an end to head checking as a way to decrease concussions in hockey deserves some attention.

Concussion in Boxing

Boxing is the one sport where one of the stated goals is to inflict a concussion (preferably with loss of consciousness) on one's opponent. This action is known, of course, as a knockout, or KO. Viewed as somewhat less impressive is the infliction of sufficient blows to induce a state of diminished cerebral arousal, which renders an opponent incapable of defending himself. This maneuver is known as a technical knock out, or TKO. The boxer shown in figure 5.3 may be capable of delivering a G-force up to 100. In short, as Dr. Julian Bailes has commented, one of the goals in boxing is to disable an opponent's central nervous system. And, as mentioned earlier, Dr. Bailes has estimated that 1,300 boxing deaths have occurred since 1880.

Boxing has been banned in three countries (Iceland, Sweden, and Norway), but this may have been more the result of reaction to corruption and illegal behaviors associated with the sport than because of concern about the health of boxers. Medical groups that have supported a ban on boxing include the American Medical Association; the American Academy of Pediatrics; the American Academy of Neurology; the California and New York State Medical Associations; the National Medical Associations of Australia, Canada, and the United Kingdom; and the World Medical Association. Bailes (2004) in a challenge to the neurosurgical community, proposed a set of initial guidelines to increase the safety of boxers.

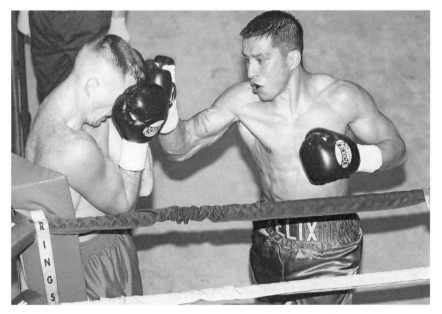

FIGURE 5.3 In boxing circles, the number of KOs and TKOs is often taken as an index of a boxer's power and strength and is often correlated positively with a boxer's ranking among peers.

Photo courtesy of Richard Riley.

- A licensed physician with special training in the early detection of neurological dysfunction be at ringside and have the authority to terminate the bout.
- The nearest hospital with neurosurgical staff should be alerted and on stand-by in the event of an injury.
- An ambulance with paramedics must be at the bout.
- Boxers must weigh in 24 hours prior to the bout to prevent dehydration procedures to meet weight requirements.
- Contestants should receive neurological examinations immediately before and after each bout by the ringside physician.

Bailes further proposed that boxers should obtain a permit in order to participate in the sport, requiring boxers to undergo a neurological examination, neuropsychological testing, an electroencephalogram (EEG), and a CT scan of the brain. These permits would have a one-year expiration date. Boxers would be required to repeat these diagnostic tests to renew the permit.

The permit to box would be similar to a passport, in that a photograph and other identifying information is included. Further, Bailes recommended that the passport contain the athlete's medical record and boxing history, including the outcomes of all bouts and any associated medical suspensions. Any boxer placed on medical suspension would surrender his passport to the boxing authorities.

Bailes also recommended national certification of trainers, referees, judges, and ringside physicians; licensing for boxing gyms; and regular inspection of equipment. Any boxer suffering a knockout (KO) or technical knockout (TKO) would be medically suspended for 45 days. Return to competition would be allowed after the athlete's neurological evaluation, EEG, and brain MRI return to normal. If an athlete sustains three consecutive TKOs or KOs, his permit would be revoked.

In 1993, Dr. Barry Jordan wrote, "Chronic traumatic brain injury (CTBI) is the most serious public health concern in modern day boxing" (p. 136, Jordan et al. 1997). CTBI is now superseding the terms *dementia pugilistica* and *chronic traumatic encephalopathy* as the standard term used to describe the cumulative neurologic consequences of repetitive head trauma in boxers. According to Jordan and colleagues, CTBI is characterized by a varied constellation of cognitive impairments, parkinsonism (motor deficits), ataxia (balance disturbances), and behavioral changes.

Early studies of boxers (pre-1980s) suggested that the multiple, subconcussive blows (impacts below the threshold to cause a concussion) experienced by boxers, along with the cumulative effects of multiple concussions, led to the "punch-drunk syndrome." However, the major view at that time was that this syndrome was relatively rare and affected only vulnerable boxers who were poorly trained, had limited education, or had problems with substance abuse (or some combination thereof). Roberts (1969) estimated that 17% of retired professional boxers suffer from CTBI. That estimated figure escalated to about 87% in a study reported by Dr. Ira Casson and associates in the *Journal of the American Medical Association* (1984).

In the 1990s, however, studies indicated that an amateur boxing status (as opposed to professional) and lowered numbers of boxing bouts were associated with less evidence of impairment on formal neuropsychological tests. Indeed, Drs. Meheroz Rabadi and Barry Jordan (2001) considered amateur boxing status as a low-risk factor for the development of CTBI. These findings began to call into question the conventional wisdom of pervasive CTBI in all boxers.

Matser and colleagues (2000) published a study of amateur boxers in *The Physician and Sportsmedicine*. Thirty eight amateur Dutch boxers were compared with 28 amateur Dutch boxing control subjects on a battery of neuropsychological tests administered before and within 20 minutes after a bout (the control group engaged in an equivalent amount of time punching a bag). All boxers wore protective headgear, per Dutch Boxing Federation regulations. Significant group differences were found on 6 of the 13 neuropsychological test scores, with control subjects outperforming the boxers on measures of planning, attention, and memory. No significant differences were found between the groups on measures of speed of information processing and attention.

Conversely, Porter (2003) reported on a prospective, 9-year neuropsychological study of 20 randomly selected actively competing male amateur boxers (in Dublin, Ireland) and 20 age- and socioeconomically matched control subjects. The results indicated no deterioration in neuropsychological test performances of the amateur boxers over the study period. It may well be the case that the immediate neurocognitive deficits noted in the Matser et al. (2000) study were temporary impairments.

In 1997 Dr. Jordan and his associates published a study of professional boxers in the *Journal of the American Medical Association*.

Although the subject size was small, the results of the study were of sufficient importance to merit an in-depth discussion. Jordan and his colleagues began with the observation that pathology studies revealed many similarities between CTBI and Alzheimer's disease (AD), including neurofibrillary tangles (shown in figure 5.4), beta-amyloid plaques, and decreased amounts of the neurotransmitter acetylcholine. They further observed that researchers had previously identified the apolipoprotein E epsilon-4 (ApoE e4) allele as a gene associated with Alzheimer's, and that head trauma was now being considered a major environmental risk factor for the development of AD. They decided to do a study assessing the potential role of this gene in the development of CTBI in boxers.

Thirty professional boxers (24 volunteer and 6 referred) ranging in age from 23 to 76 were examined with a detailed neurological examination; cognitive testing (summed as a CBI composite, or chronic brain injury score); ApoE-e4 genotyping; and medical, social, family, and boxing histories. The average age was 49, and 27 of the 30 boxers were retired. Eleven were Caucasian, 10 were African American, and 9 were Hispanic. Boxing exposure was clas-

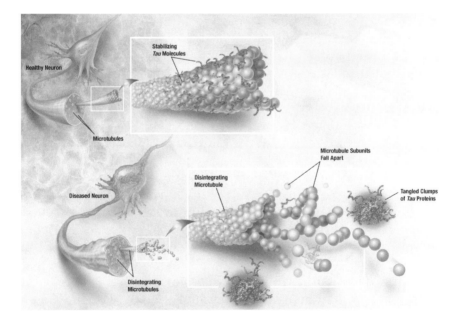

FIGURE 5.4   Neurofibrillary tangles.

Courtesy of the Alzheimer's Disease Education and Referral Center, a service of the National Institute on Aging.

sified as high or low based on a previous study, which showed that an average of 12 bouts best differentiated the two groups.

Nineteen of the 30 boxers (63%) exhibited abnormalities on the cognitive tests. High-exposure boxers (more than 12 bouts) had worse cognitive scores than low-exposure boxers. Twelve boxers (40% of the sample) were considered to have mild CTBI, 4 (13%) had moderate CTBI, and 3 (10%) had severe CTBI. The remaining 11 boxers were classified as having normal CTBI scores. The 3 boxers classified as having severe CTBI all had at least one copy of ApoE e4. Two of the 4 boxers with moderate CTBI (50%) were positive for the gene, and 3 of the 12 boxers (25%) with mild CTBI tested positive for ApoE e4. Only 2 of the 11 boxers with normal CTBI scores (18%) were positive for the gene.

When the boxers were assessed in terms of boxing exposure, it was found that those boxers with high exposure *and* the ApoE-e4 allele had cognitive scores that were twice as poor as high-exposure boxers *without* the ApoE-e4 allele. Low-exposure boxers (with or without the ApoE-e4 allele) had the best cognitive test scores. The authors concluded that this preliminary study suggested that the ApoE-e4 allele "may predispose a boxer to developing CTBI, especially in those with high exposure to the sport." (p. 139)

Rabadi and Jordan, in their 2001 article in the *Clinical Journal of Sport Medicine,* noted the following risk factors for the development of CTBI in boxers: professional status, retirement after the age of 28, boxing longer than 10 years, and participating in more than 150 bouts. Suspected risk factors included increased sparring exposure, previous TKO or KO, poor boxing performance, being a nonscientific slugger who was difficult to knock out, and possibly ApoE e4 genotype. In a similar vein, Dr. Lisa Ravdin and her associates published a study of boxers in the *Clinical Journal of Sport Medicine* (2003). They found in their study of 26 boxers that those who had the highest boxing exposure (again defined as more than 12 professional bouts) had the poorest memory-test performances on a battery of neuropsychological tests.

Moriarity and colleagues (2004) reported on a prospective, controlled study of 82 collegiate amateur boxers participating in a 7-day, single-elimination tournament. Control subjects were 30 matched nonboxing participants. Cognitive functioning was evaluated with CogSport (a computer-based platform of cognitive tests) both before the tournament and within 2 hours of the completion of each bout. Boxers whose bout was stopped by the referee showed slowed responses on reaction-time tasks. On measures of simple and choice reaction times and working memory, there were no group differences between those boxers who completed one, two, or three bouts. The authors concluded, "With the exception of boxers whose contest is stopped by the referee, amateur boxers participating in multiple bouts during a 7-day tournament display no evidence of cognitive dysfunction in the immediate postbout period" (p. 1497).

We were hesitant to discuss boxing in this book because we believe that this sport may stand alone in terms of risk to the brain (cycling not included). Blows to the head in boxing (in sparring and in bouts) may far outweigh, both qualitatively and quantitatively, any impacts to the head received in any other sport. We also suspect that the cumulative effects of boxing are very different from those noted in other sports.

So, if you're a boxer, should you run out to your family doctor and ask for ApoE testing? Probably not. ApoE testing is not perfectly predictive of who will develop Alzheimer's disease (on the average, ApoE testing may be only 67% correct in determining Alzheimer's). Instead, if you're in boxing, perhaps the best thing to do is to limit your number of bouts. According to the current numbers, participating in 12 professional bouts before age 28 appears to be pushing the envelope.

Concussion in Soccer

Soccer is one of the oldest games in the world, with references to the game noted in ancient Chinese (200 B.C.) and Greek (4 B.C.) writings. It is the most popular sport in the world, with an estimated 120 million players worldwide, including 16 million in the United States (Putukian 2004). It is probably the fastest growing team sport in the United States, especially among women.

A unique aspect of soccer is the purposeful use of the unprotected head for controlling and advancing the ball, called "heading" the ball (shown in figure 5.5). The NCAA reported that collegiate soccer players have the highest rate of concussions among players of organized contact sports that do not involve the use of helmets. The burning question in soccer at present is whether heading the ball leads to brain injury. In this section we will discuss concussions in soccer and the available information on heading and possible cerebral injury.

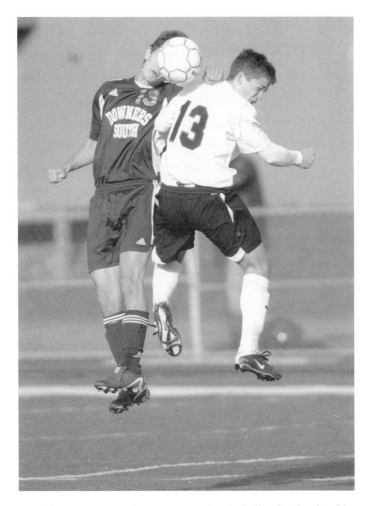

FIGURE 5.5 When two soccer players compete for the ball, a head-to-head impact could occur.

© Human Kinetics.

In a 1994 text, Dr. R.W. Dick reported a concussion incidence of 0.25 per 1,000 athletic exposures (AE) in male soccer players and a rate of 0.24 for female soccer players. Other recent studies have shown concussion rates ranging from 0.14 to 0.60 per 1,000 AE for men and 0.15 to 0.40 per 1,000 AE for women. Studies have shown that anywhere from 25% to more than 40% of soccer athletes have sustained a concussion by the end of their high school career. Among collegiate soccer athletes, 12 to 13% acknowledge having had a concussion in the prior season, and as many as 63%

will admit to having had signs and symptoms of a concussion in the prior season (Delaney et al. 2001, 2002). Undoubtedly, concussion occurs frequently in soccer.

How do these concussions occur? Drs. John Powell and K.D. Barber-Foss, in a 1999 article in the *Journal of the American Medical Association,* found that 59% of soccer concussions occurred as a result of player-to-player contact while heading the ball, with 30.5% occurring as a result of other (nonheading) player-to-player contact. Concussions also resulted from contact with goal posts and the ground.

The Federation of International Football Associations (FIFA) Medical Assessment and Research Center studied 398 soccer matches, reflecting 10,155 hours of soccer play. Head injuries accounted for about 15% of all injuries. Fourteen concussions were reported, and all were due to head-to-head contact and not due to heading the ball. The rates of concussion vary because of a wide array of factors, including inconsistent definitions and diagnosis of concussion, the questionable accuracy of athletes' self-diagnosis and memory of concussion, and possible underreporting of concussion by athletes. The rates also may vary as a function of amount of competition; the more an athlete competes, the greater the chance for a concussion. Gender differences may also be a relevant factor, as a study by Covassin and colleagues (2003) revealed that female NCAA soccer players sustained more concussions per game than their male counterparts.

The primary question about heading the ball is whether the repeated subconcussive blows incurred while heading the ball in soccer is analogous to the multiple blows received in boxing, thus leading to an impairment in and possible degeneration of cerebral functioning. Put more quaintly, do the "dings" lead to dementia? (Credit goes to Dr. Jeff Barth of the University of Virginia for the "dings to dementia" quip.)

The first mention of the issue of soccer-related effects to the head was in 1972 in the *British Journal of Sport Medicine.* In that article, Dr. W.B. Mathews coined the term "footballer's migraine," referring to the postcompetition painful headaches experienced by many soccer players. Since that time, a wide array of studies has appeared, assessing symptoms, neuropsychological test performances, and neuroimaging results in soccer athletes. Let's take a look at some of these findings.

Symptoms

Numerous studies have documented acute and chronic symptoms among active and retired soccer athletes. The most frequently reported symptoms include headache, neck pain, dizziness, irritability, poor concentration, and a sense of being dazed. One study has shown that headers report more headache than nonheaders. Headache seems to be the most frequently reported symptom in those who head the ball regularly.

Electroencephalographic (EEG) Studies

EEGs are electrical recordings of brain activity made by attaching surface electrodes to the scalp. EEGs are utilized in the assessment of abnormal electrical activity in the brain and are used primarily in the diagnosis of seizure disorders. A series of studies (mostly by Tysvaer and associates) appeared in the 1980s and early 1990s looking at possible EEG abnormalities in soccer players. Three studies showed no significant EEG abnormalities in headers versus nonheaders, and one study showed no significant differences in EEGs between retired soccer players and control subjects. To date, no compelling evidence has been found that heading the ball in soccer leads to EEG abnormalities.

CT and MRI Studies

Several studies have looked for differences in brain structure in soccer athletes. Sortland and Tysvaer (1989) found atrophy (shrinkage) of the brain on CT (computed axial tomography) scans in retired professional Scandinavian soccer athletes. The authors found that atrophy was greater for the headers. Unfortunately, no control subjects were used in the study, and the headers (as a group) were older than the nonheaders. This factor is important because, as we discussed in the section on basic brain facts, some degree of atrophy occurs as a function of aging. Therefore, it is unclear whether the atrophy was due to heading, concussions, aging, or some interaction among the variables.

Two studies of soccer athletes (Haglund and Eriksson 1993; Jordan et al. 1996) found no brain magnetic resonance imaging (MRI) differences between soccer athletes and appropriate control subjects. At present, like the EEG, there is no convincing evidence that heading the ball in soccer leads to brain abnormalities as detected by standard CT or MRI.

Immediate Effects

Studies have addressed the immediate performance consequences of heading the ball in soccer on the EEG, cognitive functioning, and balance. An early study (Koss 1983) found that 2 of 10 soccer athletes had an abnormal EEG after 15 minutes of header training. No control subjects were used in this study. More recent studies have shown no adverse effects on neuropsychological test performance between headers and nonheaders after 20 minutes of header training (Putukian et al. 2001), 10 games (Putukian, Echemendia, et al. 2001), and an entire season (reported by Echemendia in Institute of Medicine 2002). Broglio and associates (2004) found no adverse effect of either linear or rotational heading on postural stability (balance testing) in collegiate soccer athletes. These studies indicate that there is no clear relationship between heading the ball and short-term neuropsychological and balance functions.

Neuropsychological Studies

One study has shown at least mild impairment on neuropsychological tests in soccer players versus control subjects (Tysvaer et al. 1991), and another has shown impairment on one of four neuropsychological tests in soccer players versus swimmers (Downs and Abwender 2002). Two studies found no differences between soccer players (who were headers) versus control subjects (Haglund and Eriksson 1993; Rasmussen et al. 2002). Guskiewicz and colleagues (2002) found no difference between collegiate soccer athletes and student controls on neuropsychological test performance (or SAT scores).

A series of three studies from the Netherlands by Dr. Erik Matser and colleagues (1998 to 2001) has appeared in several journals and merits further scrutiny. In the first study (published in the journal *Neurology*, 1998), the authors compared 53 active professional Dutch soccer players with 27 elite track and swimming athletes (control subjects) on cognitive tests of memory, planning, and visuoperceptual functioning. Generally speaking, the soccer players performed poorer on the tests than the control athletes. An inverse correlation was found between neuropsychological test scores and the combination of number of soccer concussions and frequency of heading the ball. In other words, the greater the number of concussions and headers, the worse the neuropsychological test scores.

The second study (published in the *Journal of the American Medical Association,* 1999) compared 33 Dutch amateur soccer players with 27 elite track and swimming athletes on 16 different neuropsychological tests. Soccer players performed more poorly on three of the neuropsychological tests than the control athletes. The authors found that the number of concussions was inversely related to neuropsychological test scores. Heading was not assessed. These results are tempered, however, by the fact that nearly 82% (27 out of 33) of the soccer players had sustained nonsoccer concussions, as opposed to 52% of the control athletes (14 out of 27). Furthermore, the soccer players averaged 50 alcoholic drinks per month versus an average of 28 for the track and swimming athletes. The possible confounding of these results because of inequality between the groups in the number of alcoholic drinks and number of concussions may need to be considered when interpreting the conclusions of this study.

The third Matser study was published in the *Journal of Clinical and Experimental Neuropsychology* in 2001. The authors studied 84 active Dutch professional soccer players and assessed the number of professional soccer concussions, the number of headers in the prior season, and neuropsychological test scores (no controls were used in this study). They found that the number of concussions was inversely related to three neuropsychological test scores, and the number of headers was inversely related to four different neuropsychological test scores. The authors acknowledged, however, that research methodology and statistical factors might have limited the findings of their study.

The Matser studies point out the research difficulties in directly assessing the effects of heading the ball on cognitive test performance. First, the effects of concussion versus heading cannot be separated out neatly. Second, it is important to consider the number of soccer- and nonsoccer-related concussions. Third, other potential influences (for example, alcohol consumption) need to be taken into account. This is just a partial list of variables that need to be considered when doing this kind of research. We give credit to Matser and his colleagues and view their studies as valuable. It's much easier to point out the shortcomings of a scientific study than to do the study itself.

Summary Reviews

Kirkendall and Garrett (2001) published a literature review of the effects of heading the ball in soccer. Their review covered the years

1965 to 2001. They concluded, "It is difficult to blame purposeful heading for the reported cognitive deficits. . . . Concussions are a common head injury in soccer (mostly from head-to-head or head-to-ground impact) and a factor in cognitive deficits and are probably the mechanism of the reported dysfunction" (p. 328).

It is important to mention a conference held in 2002 by the Institute of Medicine. The conference was titled "Is Soccer Bad for Children's Heads?" Leading national experts presented at the conference. The conclusion of the conference was that "To date, there has been no published study that has provided direct evidence that the practice of heading a soccer ball causes long-term deficits in mental function." They hastened to add, however, "Nor has any study been published that proves heading has no long-term effects." The conference results are available on line; see appendix B for the link. It is also noteworthy that McCrory (2004) questioned whether concussion guidelines for adults should be used with children, or whether separate guidelines for children were needed.

Dr. Margot Putukian (2004) (now at Princeton University) concluded, "Although it appears that heading in soccer is safe, it does appear that concussions occur commonly, and that these injuries, if severe or multiple, may be of concern" (p. 13). Some sports medicine clinicians have suggested that it is not heading per se that leads to cognitive dysfunction in soccer players, but it is the behavior of heading (Witol and Webbe 2003) or ". . . the act of going up to challenge for a ball . . ." (Putukian 2004, p.13) that leads to concussion and the resulting adverse cognitive effects.

Finally, several case reports have been published in the *British Journal of Sports Medicine* (Demetriades et al. 2004) raising questions about the safety of heading the ball for athletes who have an arachnoid cyst. An arachnoid cyst occurs in the brain, usually as the result of a developmental abnormality. The cyst is thought to result from an abnormal duplication or splitting of the arachnoid membrane and is thus typically congenital in nature. Arachnoid cysts of the middle fossa (a channel in the middle part of the brain) occur more commonly in males (4:1 ratio versus females). The cysts are usually asymptomatic and are most frequently discovered as an incidental finding when a patient undergoes a brain scan. Dr. Demetriades and colleagues reported a case of a 24-year-old university student (with a reputation for being a frequent "header") who developed a subdural hematoma after competition. The athlete denied any history of head trauma, but during questioning acknowledged having headaches and feeling slightly lightheaded after twice-weekly practices. The symptoms were said to subside slowly during the 24 hours after practice. The patient came to medical attention after 6 weeks of increasing nausea and headache, unsteadiness, mild right-sided weakness, and 2 days of vomiting. CT scan of the brain revealed a large subdural hematoma lying superficial to a left middle-fossa arachnoid cyst. The athlete underwent successful neurosurgical evacuation of the hematoma; clinical recovery was said to be satisfactory and without residual neurological deficit.

Demetriades and colleagues discuss in their article the potential danger of contact competition for athletes with known arachnoid cysts, and they cite three other similar cases of subdural hematoma in athletes with arachnoid cysts. This is a clear instance of the potentially deleterious effects of heading the soccer ball in specifically vulnerable individuals. We view these cases as exceptions, rather than the rule, because the actual number of athletes with symptomatically silent arachnoid cysts is unknown. As the authors point out, it would not be cost effective to have every athlete undergo a CT scan of the head prior to competition. Demetriades and his associates do caution sports medicine physicians that a "protracted history but consistently linked to repetitive head injury should alert the physician to the possibility of an arachnoid cyst" (e8, p. 2). To this we would add male gender as a specific risk factor, since the patients involved in the reported studies have all been male, and the gender ratio for arachnoid cysts of the middle fossa is 4:1 in favor of males.

We are in agreement with Kirkendall and Garrett (2001), who concluded,

> It is difficult to blame purposeful heading for the reported cognitive deficits when actual heading exposure and details of the nature of head-ball impacts are unknown. Concussions are a common head injury in soccer (mostly from head-head or head-ground impact) and a factor in cognitive deficits and are probably the mechanism of the reported dysfunction. (p. 328)

We await the results of prospective studies regarding the possible relationship(s) among playing soccer, heading the ball, sustaining concussions, and cognitive functioning.

A review of the literature on heading the ball in soccer indicates that those athletes most likely to display abnormal brain functioning (either on brain imaging measures or neuropsychological tests) are retired Scandinavian soccer players. We suspect that this is the case for several reasons. First, many of these athletes competed when the soccer ball used was covered in leather. Leather absorbs water and can increase the mass of a soccer ball by 20%. The soccer balls used in competition today are not covered in leather and therefore do not absorb water. It is possible that the wet leather balls used in the 1960s and 1970s generated greater physical force than the balls used currently and thus were more of a concussive risk. Second, the moderator variables of player alcohol and drug use, age, native intellect, and other concussion history may all be relevant, independently and/or in combination. Third, inflated ball pressure, goal-post protection (or lack thereof), type of turf, and other environmental factors may also come into play here. In short, the perfect study on concussion in soccer has yet to be done.

Research Digest

NFL concussion studies (Pellman et al. 2003a-b, 2004a-c, 2005):

There were 887 concussions (games and practices) from a total of 650 athletes in the NFL study; 787 (89%) of the concussions occurred in games. In the laboratory reconstructions of concussion in the NFL, the lowest peak head acceleration was to the facemask (78 plus or minus 18 g) versus an average of 107 to 117 g for impacts elsewhere. Concussed players averaged 3.7 plus or minus 2.7 initial signs and symptoms. The relative risk (RR) for concussion by position (the ratio is concussions per game to position) is quarterback 1.62, wide receiver 1.23, tight end 0.94, and defensive backs 0.93. The RR for concussion by type of play (the ratio is numbers of concussions per 1,000 plays) is kickoff (9.29%), punt returns (3.86%), rushing plays (2.24%), and passing plays (2.14%).

The most common clinical symptoms immediately postconcussion were headache (55%), dizziness (41.8%), and blurred vision (16.3%). The most common clinical signs noted on physical examination immediately postconcussion were problems with immediate recall (25.5%), retrograde amnesia (18%), and information-processing problems (17.5%).

One hundred and sixty (24.6%) athletes experienced a repeat concussion during the study (1996-2001); 51 of the 160 (7.8% of the total) sustained 3 or more concussions, and 72 concussions (8.1% of the total) led to an athlete being taken out of play for 7 or more days. The highest frequency of athletes missing more than 7 days due to concussion (by position) were quarterbacks (14.8%), the return unit on special teams (11.8%), and defensive backs (10.8%). Lovell and Barr (2004) present a more general overview of the use of neuropsychological testing in the NFL.

Soccer studies:

Jordan et al. (1996), in a study of NCAA soccer athletes, reported a concussion rate of 0.14 per 1,000 AE for men and 0.15 per 1,000 AE for women. Boden et al. (1998), in a 2-year study of elite Atlantic Coast Conference soccer athletes, found a concussion rate of 0.6 per 1,000 AE for men and a rate of 0.4 per 1,000 AE for women.

In a study of 1,659 children ages 7 to 13 in the Pittsburgh area, Radelet and associates (2002) found a concussion incidence of 0.21 per 1,000 AE over two seasons. Kirkendall and Garrett (2001) found that head injuries accounted for 15% of the soccer injuries incurred by 12- to 18-year-olds.

Echemendia (1997) reported that 41.2% of male and 42.2% of female incoming freshmen soccer athletes had sustained at least one concussion in their high school careers. In the Institute for Medicine's "Is Soccer Bad for Children's Heads?" (2002), Brooks found that more than 25% of soccer high school athletes had experienced at least one concussion. The studies by Delaney et al. (2001, 2002) found that collegiate soccer athletes who had a prior history of concussion were 3 to 11 times more likely to have had a concussion than those players who had never had a concussion. Also, collegiate soccer women were 2.5 times more likely to sustain a concussion than their male counterparts.

The specific neuropsychological test in which the soccer athletes in the Downs and Abwender study (2002) performed more poorly was the Wisconsin Card Sorting Test.

Barnes et al. (1998) found that 18% of the concussions found among collegiate athletes were due to the use of incorrect techniques when heading the ball.

The Guskiewicz et al. (2002) study involved 240 Division I NCAA athletes, including 91 soccer players, 96 female lacrosse/field hockey and baseball players, and 53 student nonathlete controls. Nearly half (49.5%) of the soccer players, 29.2% of the nonsoccer athletes, and 15.2% of the student controls reported a positive concussion history.

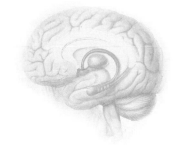

chapter 6

Current Trends, Research, and the Future

In this chapter we review the efforts being directed toward sport concussion by various medical organizations. We address the possible cumulative effects of concussion, the question of how many concussions are too many, and the potential long-term effects of concussion. We also discuss the role of helmets and what can be done about concussion.

What Are Professional Organizations Doing About Sport Concussion?

The 1990s saw an explosion of assessment protocols, grading scales, and return-to-play (RTP) criteria for sport concussion. It is worthwhile to take a careful look at some of the more frequently used systems in an attempt to discern their similarities and differences.

The most recent and currently recommended management system came out of the First International Conference on Sport Concussion, held in Vienna, Austria, in 2001. The conference was sponsored by the IIHF (International Ice Hockey Federation), the FIFA (Federation of International Football Associations), and the IOC (International Olympic Committee). This group has come to be known as the Concussion in Sport (CIS) Group. It is worthwhile to note that some members and authors of the document are also the authors of the most widely used concussion grading systems. The major recommendations, which were published in 2002 and first used at the 2001 Olympics, are summarized here:

- No particular grading scale is recommended.
- Sideline assessment and neuropsychological testing are recommended.
- An athlete may return to play when the athlete is asymptomatic at rest and with exertion, the neuropsychological test scores (if baseline testing has been done) have returned to baseline, the graduated rehabilitation program has been completed, and medical clearance has been given by the attending physician.

For the full report, see CIS Group (2002). We consider this report to be required reading for sports medicine clinicians interested in concussion.

In November 2004 the Second International Symposium on Concussion in Sport was held in Prague, endorsed again by FIFA, IIHF, and IOC. A key group of leaders in the field of sport concussion were brought together to update concussion research and management topics, modeling the meeting after that held in Vienna in 2001. A consensus document was again copublished and appeared in the April 2005 issues of *The Physician and Sportsmedicine, British Journal of Sports Medicine,* and the *Clinical Journal of Sport Medicine.*

New concepts from that meeting include the descriptions of concussion as either simple (resolving in about a week) or complex (lasting longer, having recurrent or persistent signs or symptoms). Details of concussion rehabilitation including sport psychology issues were reviewed and the importance of neuropsychological testing was partially reinforced. The new concept of cognitive (mental) exertion as an aggravating factor for persistent symptoms was explored, particularly in the pediatric age groups. This concept refers to the fact that sustained mental activity and effort, in a manner similar to physical exertion, can worsen the symptoms of concussion in recently concussed athletes. In addition, although the Vienna guidelines were seen to be applicable to concussion in children, the important unique features in children were emphasized and the call for more research in that age group identified. Agreement exists that a conservative approach is mandated in childhood sport concussion.

The National Athletic Trainers' Association (NATA) has published a position statement on the management of sport-related concussion (Guskiewicz et al. 2004). It is a comprehensive document, and one that we also consider required reading for sports medicine clinicians and ATCs in particular. The document is organized into major sections including Defining and Recognizing Concussion, Evaluating and Making Return-to-Play Decisions, Concussion Assessment Tools, When to Refer an Athlete to a Physician After a Concussion, When to Disqualify an Athlete, Special Considerations for the Younger Athlete, Home Care, and Equipment Issues. The NATA position statement is well documented and essentially recommends the use of baseline testing for all athletes, including clinical symptoms, mental status, balance assessment, and neuropsychological functioning. The recommendations are constructed in a way that offers flexibility for baseline and postconcussion assessment given an individual team's professional and financial resources.

The criteria for disqualifying a concussed athlete from same-day participation are specific, and emphasis is placed appropriately on the more conservative management of younger athletes. The appendices contain a concussion-symptom scale, a physician-referral checklist, and an excellent "Concussion Home Instructions" guide. The NATA position statement is the most detailed and specific management guidelines for sport concussion ever published.

One recent addition is the position paper published in the *Clinical Journal of Sport Medicine* (2005) by the Concussion in Rodeo Group, based on the first international research and clinical care conference held in Calgary July 7 through 9, 2004.

Previously, numerous other professional organizations have developed standards for sport concussion. As you examine these, keep in mind that the grading of concussion is tied to RTP criteria. Here are some examples:

- The Canadian Academy of Sport Medicine Concussion Committee (CASM): In 2000, CASM published assessment and RTP guidelines in the *Clinical Journal of Sport Medicine.* No grading system for concussion was endorsed or recommended. An athlete manifesting any symptoms of concussion should not RTP during that contest. RTP criteria were based on a stepwise rehabilitative program after resolution of all symptoms, at rest and with exertion. Indeed, the RTP criteria adopted by the CIS Group (previously discussed) were essentially derived from those recommended by the CASM.

• American Orthopedic Society for Sports Medicine (AOSSM): The findings of the Concussion Workshop, sponsored by AOSSM, were published in *The American Journal of Sports Medicine* (Wojtys et al. 1999). This group offered recommendations for initial assessment of the concussed athlete and RTP guidelines but did not offer a grading system for concussion. AOSSM guidelines for RTP are divided into "Return to Play (Same Day)" and "Delayed Return to Play (Not the Same Day)" classifications. The AOSSM guidelines state that an athlete with any LOC is not to RTP during that contest. Athletes sustaining a concussion should be monitored closely for a minimum of 15 minutes. If the athlete has symptoms that abate within 15 minutes (at rest and with exertion), has a normal neurological evaluation, and did not lose consciousness, the athlete may RTP in that contest. Signs or symptoms lasting for more than 15 minutes preclude RTP during that contest.

• American Academy of Neurology (AAN): The AAN's Quality Standards Subcommittee published "Practice Parameter: The Management of Concussion in Sports" in *Neurology* (1997), offering a grading scale and RTP criteria for sport concussion. A Grade 1 concussion was defined as transient confusion, no LOC, and concussion symptoms or mental-status abnormalities on examination resolving within 15 minutes. A concussed athlete should be checked every 5 minutes. An athlete may RTP if concussion symptoms and mental status abnormalities have cleared within 15 minutes. However, a second Grade 1 concussion within the same contest eliminates that player from competition that day, with the player returning only if asymptomatic at rest and with exertion for 1 week.

A Grade 2 concussion was defined as transient confusion, no LOC, and concussion symptoms or mental-status abnormalities on examination lasting more than 15 minutes. Any persistent Grade 2 symptoms lasting for more than 1 hour warrant medical attention. An athlete with a Grade 2 concussion may not RTP in that contest. The athlete should be monitored closely that day and examined by a trained person the following day. A physician should perform a neurological examination to clear the athlete for RTP after 1 full asymptomatic week at rest and with exertion. Continuation of symptoms for more than a week may necessitate CT or MRI scanning. For an athlete with a second Grade 2 concussion, RTP should be deferred until 2 weeks of no symptoms at rest and with exertion.

A Grade 3 concussion was defined as any LOC, either brief (seconds) or prolonged (minutes). If serious clinical signs are noted, the athlete should be transported via ambulance to the nearest emergency department where a thorough neurological examination should be performed. Neuroimaging studies and hospital admission may be indicated. In the case of an athlete discharged from the emergency room, neurological status should be checked daily until symptoms have stabilized or resolved.

The AAN system mandates removal from play for 1 week after multiple Grade 1 concussions. RTP is withheld for 1 week after a Grade 2 concussion, and for 2 weeks after multiple Grade 2 concussions. Grade 3 concussion (brief LOC) mandates 1 week on the sideline, while Grade 3 (prolonged LOC) leads to 2 weeks of not playing. Multiple Grade 3 concussions lead to withholding an athlete from play for 1 month or longer, based on the clinical decision of the treating physician.

Keep in mind that all of these time restrictions in the AAN system are based from the point where the athlete is free of symptoms, both at rest and after exertion. For example, if an athlete sustains a Grade 2 concussion in a contest on Friday evening and continues to have a headache that does not cease until the following Monday, the athlete cannot RTP for 7 days from that Monday. Time held out of competition is determined not by the date of the concussion but by the date of the resolution of all symptoms, at rest and with exertion.

It is impressive to see these groups taking concussion seriously and recognizing its potential dangers. The establishment of grading scales and RTP criteria has been a worthy pursuit, yet the divergent final products attest to how truly difficult it is to accomplish these endeavors. What appears most attractive about the CIS Group's guidelines are its multidisciplinary approach and the abandonment of medical specialty-specific guidelines for concussion evaluation and assessment. It was an attempt to get neurologists, orthopedic surgeons, neuropsychologists, athletic trainers, neurosurgeons, and all sports medicine professionals dealing with concussion on the same page. We view this as a significant step in the right direction.

What Are the Long-Term Effects of Concussion?

It is fascinating that people are shocked to hear that there may be long-term consequences to concussion. These are often the same people who are aware that athletes may have trouble with joint function, arthritis, and chronic pain after years of exposure to contact sports. They are aware that the multiple arthroscopic knee surgeries athletes undergo may take a toll down the road and that the arms, legs, knees, hips, and backs may pay a price in the future. Many never stop to realize, however, that the brain also may pay a price for exposure to repeated trauma. Dr. Julian Bailes is fond of saying that athletes are the only group of patients he knows who ask forcefully for permission to return to the opportunity for repeated exposure to head trauma.

We are just beginning to address the question of long-term effects of sport concussion so the answers are sparse at present. However, some very good scientific studies of the long-term effects of head injury in the *general population* are appearing in the literature. Current research in the general population indicates that certain types of concussion may result in an increased risk for Alzheimer's Disease (AD) and major depression. Because much has been made about these studies in the popular press, it will be worthwhile to take a closer look at them in the following sections. It is important to remember that these are not studies of sport concussion but of head injury in the general population; we cannot assume that these results are generalizable to athletes.

Alzheimer's Disease

Alzheimer's disease (AD) is a degenerative disease of the brain. It was named after the German physician Alois Alzheimer who published the first case study of the disease in 1907. The disease involves the systematic destruction of brain cells as a result of the development of beta-amyloid plaques (a derivative of the naturally occurring amyloid precursor protein found outside of nerve cells that form the basis of plaques, which are sticky aggregations of abnormal cells) and the tangling of nerve cells (neurofibrillary tangles) that occur after disruption of the normal tau protein process (tau is a protein that helps to maintain the structure of key components in nerve cells). Figure 6.1 compares PET scans of a brain with AD and a normal brain. AD is irreversible and is progressive in nature. Drugs exist to slow down the process, but as of yet, there is no cure.

The 1990s yielded research connecting concussion and head injury with the development of AD. Neuropsychologist Brenda Plassman and her colleagues (2000) examined the association between early adult head injury and the presence of dementia later in life. Dementia is a group of diseases of the brain, often degenerative in nature, of which AD is the most common. Plassman and her associates evaluated the military records of World War II navy and marine veterans who were treated for nonpenetrating (closed) head injuries. World War II soldiers who were hospitalized for the treatment of pneumonia or laceration, puncture, or incision wounds served as controls in the study. The authors reviewed military medical records of the World War II veterans to abstract the details of the closed head injuries. The entire sample was then evaluated in a multistage procedure to screen for dementia and AD.

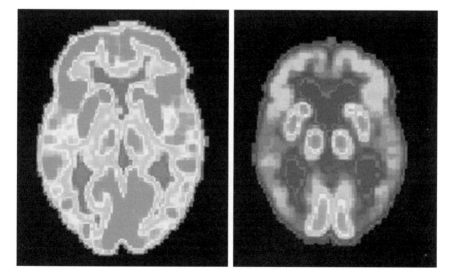

FIGURE 6.1 Alzheimer's disease causes decreased metabolism in the brain (right), as can be seen in this PET scan when compared to a normal brain (left).

Courtesy of the Alzheimer's Disease Education and Referral Center, a service of the National Institute on Aging.

The results were startling. Overall, having any type of head injury doubled a veteran's odds of developing AD, and more than doubled it for any type of dementia. The risk for AD and dementia increased with the severity of the head injury (those classified as moderate or severe). The mild head injury group, however, showed no significant risk of AD or dementia when compared with the control group of veterans with no history of head injuries.

Dr. Plassman and her researchers concluded, "The observed dose-response pattern may support a causal effect of head injury in the pathogenesis of AD and dementia" (p. 1164). In other words, the results of the Plassman study suggest that the more severe the ("dose" of) head injury, the greater the risk for the later development of dementia or AD. We emphasize the words "may support."

Dr. Z. Guo and associates (2000) published another study relevant to this issue in the journal *Neurology*. This study was designed to assess the relationship between head injury and AD. The results were truly surprising. Head injury with LOC increased the risk for AD by a factor of 9.9 (nearly a 10-fold increase), and head injury without LOC increased the risk for AD by a factor of 3.1 (a three-fold increase). Analysis by gender indicated a higher risk for AD in men with head injuries than in women with head injuries.

The two studies just described indicate that if one has a moderate or severe head injury, an injury that includes LOC or prolonged posttraumatic amnesia (probably of 30 minutes or longer), a head injury may increase one's chances of developing AD. The data for mild head injury has been less convincing. However, a recent study (Sundstrom et al. 2004) points to the presence of the ApoE gene as a potential culprit in cognitive functions post head injury, even after a mild head injury.

What is missing in the sports medicine literature is a longitudinal neuropsychological and ApoE genotyping study of *athletes* who experience a concussion or multiple mild concussions over a period of time. We doubt, however, that the data in that study (whenever it is published) will be very encouraging. There is certainly no evidence that concussions are good for one's health.

Major Depression

According to the American Psychiatric Association's *Diagnostic and Statistical Manual of Mental Disorders* (1994), the symptoms of major depression include depressed mood, loss of interest in and pleasure from daily activities, weight loss or gain, disturbed sleep pattern, fatigue, feelings of worthlessness, diminished ability to think or concentrate, and recurrent thoughts of death (that could lead to suicide). Clusters of these symptoms must be present for 2 weeks before a patient meets the criteria for major depression. It is estimated that about one in seven Americans (approximately 14%) suffers from major depression.

Dr. Tracy Holsinger and colleagues (2002) addressed the relationship between head injury and the later development of depression. The participants in this study were the same World War II navy and marine corps veterans studied by Dr. Plassman and her associates (2000) in the research previously described. The exception was that any veteran with AD or dementia of any type was excluded from this study.

Lifetime prevalence of major depression was 18.5% in those with a history of closed head injury versus 13.4% in those with no head injury. Current major depression was detected in 11.2% of the head-injured veterans versus 8.5% of the veterans without head injury. Data provided in other research has indicated about a 9.6% to 12.7% prevalence rate of depression in adult males in the United States (Koenig et al. 1999; Steffens et al. 2000), which is about the same rate noted in the control group of veterans in the Holsinger study. Interestingly, Holsinger and colleagues noted that when the head injury was categorized as mild, moderate, or severe, the results again suggest a dose-response relationship between head injury and the development of depression. In essence, the presence of a history of head injury increased a veteran's odds of developing major depression later in life by a factor of about 1.5.

Now let's take a look at a study involving athletes with head injuries and the possible development of AD and major depression. Dr. Julian Bailes and colleagues conducted a survey study of over 2,500 retired NFL players, which was presented at the 2003 American Association of Neurological Surgeons (Bailes et al. 2003). Their results indicated that NFL players who sustained three or four concussions during their career were twice as likely to develop major depression later in life as those who had not had a concussion. NFL players who had five or more concussions were nearly three times as likely to develop clinical depression later in life, suggesting a linear, dose-response relationship between concussion and later-life onset clinical depression. Dr. Bailes reported no relationship between concussion and the development of either stroke or Alzheimer's disease among retired NFL players.

Karen Johnston and colleagues (Chen et al. 2004) have found that depression and concussion-based functional MRI abnormalities may both be present in concussed athletes. It is indeed conceivable that certain types of concussions may lead to symptoms that mimic or overlap with those of clinical depression (for example, disturbed sleep, concentration problems, mood changes). We hope that these fMRI findings will be a source of clues for future treatment.

Keep in mind that the Bailes study relied on athletes' self-diagnosis and not on formal medical examinations or even a review of medical records. Many patients who develop AD can present initially with symptoms that mimic a major depression. Many Alzheimer's experts believe that the onset of a major depressive episode in an elderly individual is heralding the beginning of AD.

We present these studies not in an attempt to frighten. Rather, we present these data so that a sports medicine professional can offer an athlete accurate information so that he or she can make an informed decision about participating (or continuing to participate) in sports. As one of us was counseling an athlete about the possible risks of returning to play too early after a concussion, the athlete calmly said, "Doc, it's always a risk out there." He was absolutely right.

How Many Concussions Are Too Many?

We have read comments by physicians in the popular press that an athlete should retire after three concussions. This recommendation is an opinion and one that is likely not based on scientific fact. The fact is that there is no magic number of how many concussions are too many or even adequate scientific information to answer this question at the present time. According to Dr. Paul McCrory (2001d), in 1945 Dr. Quigley developed the "three-strikes rule" wherein an athlete who experiences three concussions in a season is out for the season. According to McCrory, this rule was adopted by Thorndike (1952), who proposed that any athlete who experienced three concussions with LOC in a season be removed from contact sports for the remainder of the season. This rule was based on clinical experience not scientific data. However, the three-strikes rule has been retained by many sports medicine clinicians and also has been incorporated into many concussion-grading systems and RTP criteria.

We believe that most experts would agree that abnormal findings on neuroimaging, persistently abnormal neuropsychological test results, ongoing clinical signs (for example, abnormal neurological exam), or continued symptoms of concussion would preclude an athlete's return to play, regardless of the absolute number of concussions. Echemendia and Cantu (2004) have echoed these general principles.

The question of "How many is too many?" has some truly unusual aspects. One of us recalls seeing an athlete who had sustained his first concussion ever. He had no LOC and no amnesia. His neuropsychological test scores were consistently below baseline during the 6 weeks postinjury, and he continued to experience symptoms. An MRI of the brain was obtained due to the prolonged symptoms and persistently abnormal test scores. The MRI revealed a nonspecific abnormality in the subcortical white matter of the brain. On the advice of a neurologist, the athlete retired from sports in his early 20s. We have all evaluated players with a history of multiple concussions whose neuropsychological test scores have always returned to baseline, whose repeated structural brain MRIs remained normal, and whose symptoms usually dissipated after less than a week. These athletes continue to play.

Dr. Paul McCrory (2002), in addressing the issue of RTP in athletes with repeated concussive injuries, wrote, "For the most part, there are no evidence-based recommendations with which to guide the practitioner" (p. 28). McCrory discussed specifics of the "neuro-mythology" surrounding concussion in sports and argued convincingly that the rule of three concussions in a season and you're out (for the season) has no basis in scientific fact, especially in the absence of documented objective evidence of brain injury. Drs. Ruben Echemendia and Robert Cantu (2004) wrote, "Experience has taught us that there is no arbitrary number of concussions that would mandate not returning to sport" (p. 494). They also discuss the issue of when it is time to stop playing sports altogether because of concussions.

Most sports medicine clinicians will not clear a player for RTP with abnormal neuroimaging results or abnormal neuropsychological test scores or if clinical signs or symptoms persist. More alarming, though, is the pattern that emerges when small, seemingly trivial hits result in symptoms that take longer and longer to go away. This pattern may be a sign of trouble and could be a warning indicator.

Are the Effects of Multiple Concussions Cumulative?

Many sports medicine professionals say absolutely yes, while others say with equal certainty no. Invariably, professionals will point to a small group of retired professional athletes, such as boxers, and conclude that the answer is yes. Or they may point to a group of retired athletes who are functioning well as sports commentators and say the answer is no. The reality is that this question is just beginning to be addressed in the sports medicine literature.

We have taken a brief look at the data on boxers (see chapter 5), but given the multitude and magnitude of blows to the head in this sport, this group may stand on its own. It is quite unlikely that other athletes incur the same exposure to concussive blows experienced by boxers. Now let's take a look at the available information on the effects of multiple concussions in athletes (mostly football players) who are not involved in the sport of boxing.

Dr. Steve Macciocchi and colleagues (2001) reported that in collegiate football players, the cognitive consequences of two concussions did not appear to be significantly different than those of one concussion. However, they acknowledged that research methodological issues placed limitations on the interpretation of their data.

Two other studies have addressed this issue with high school athletes. Dr. Michael Collins and colleagues (2002) reported data suggestive of a cumulative effect of multiple concussions similar to data reported by Dr. Grant Iverson and colleagues (2002). Collins et al. (2002) formed two groups of high school athletes based on concussion history. The first group was composed of 60 players who had never had a concussion. The second group was composed of 28 athletes with a history of three or more concussions. Trained medical staff observed the players during the season and, after a concussion, rated the players for "on-field markers of concussion"(LOC, anterograde amnesia, retrograde amnesia, and confusion). Medical staff also noted whether the player's mental status changes lasted for less than or greater than 5 minutes. Only 9.4% of the players with no prior history of concussion experienced mental-status changes for more than 5 minutes, whereas over three times as many of the players with three or more prior concussions (31.6%) had mental-status changes lasting more than 5 minutes. Only 3.7% of the athletes with no prior concussion history displayed three of the four on-field markers of concussion, whereas 26.3% of the players with a history of three or more concussions exhibited three of the four markers.

Collins and his associates concluded that the findings might reflect a lower concussion threshold in athletes who sustain multiple concussions. They also questioned whether the players with multiple concussions were "selectively vulnerable" to the injury of concussion. The issues of genetics (for example, ApoE status) and natural endowment of basic cognitive abilities were seen as potentially relevant in these circumstances. Many studies have demonstrated an increased risk for concussion after having the first one, although other experts (see McCrory 1999) have challenged this clinical maxim.

Dr. Grant Iverson and associates (2004a) conducted a study to examine the possibility that athletes with multiple concussions might show cumulative effects. Nineteen athletes with multiple concussions (three or more) were matched carefully with 19 players with no concussion history prior to the current season. Athletes in both groups had sustained a concussion in the current season.

Iverson found that the multiple-concussion group had lower memory test scores on the Immediate Postconcussion Assessment and Cognitive Testing (ImPACT) after a concussion, reported significantly more symptoms after a concussion, and demonstrated a greater number of on-field markers of concussion than their once-concussed peers. Players with a history of multiple concussions were six times more likely to experience posttraumatic amnesia and about eight times more likely to experience five or more minutes of mental-status changes. Iverson interpreted these data as reflecting the cumulative effects of concussive injury. However, these findings also could be interpreted as reflecting an increased vulnerability to the next injury, and not a cumulative effect.

The NCAA Concussion Study also addressed this issue (Guskiewicz, McCrea, Marshall, et al. 2003). The authors studied 2,905 football players from 25 U.S. colleges during the 1999 through 2001 football seasons. Of the players studied, 184 players (6.3%) had a concussion, and 12 of these players (6.5%) sustained a repeat concussion within the same season. Players with a history of three or more prior concussions had a slower recovery rate than players with one prior concussion. Symptoms lasted for longer than 1 week in 30% of those players with three or more prior concussions compared to 14.6% of those with one prior concussion.

Dr. Ken Kutner and associates (2000) presented data on active NFL players suggesting that older players who possessed the ApoE-e4 allele performed worse on cognitive tests than younger players with or without the e4 allele. Although the number of concussions was not assessed directly in this study, the authors suggested that the age variable was a "proxy" indicator of high or low contact exposure (and presumed concussion) among the professional athletes. It should be noted that the sample size in this study was very small and that age differences may have been a major factor. Although preliminary, these findings indicate that greater attention needs to be paid to the potential role of the ApoE factor in the cognitive aspects of sport-concussion assessment and rehabilitation.

Most of the research shows that risk to have another concussion increases if you've already had one, but that depends on many other factors. For some athletes, recurrent concussions appear to cause greater symptoms, cognitive problems, and lengthier recovery time. Furthermore, our operational definitions of "cumulative" versus "increased vulnerability" are not yet clear.

Do Helmets Help?

Generally speaking, helmets have been used as a way of decreasing the probability of skull fracture resulting from linear-impact injuries to the head. Helmets are generally sport specific. Some helmets are designed for multiple collisions (football), whereas others are designed for a single, unintended collision (automobile racing). The racer in figure 6.2 is putting on this type of helmet. A number of agencies are involved in delineating standards for helmet manufacturing. Among these agencies are the Canadian Standard Association, the National Operating Committee on Safety in Athletic Equipment, the American National Standards Institute, and the American Society for Testing and Materials. Drs. John Powell and Thomas Dompier provided an excellent overview of the role of the helmet in sport-concussion prevention in a 2004 issue of *Current Sports Medicine Reports*.

According to Dr. Michael Levy and colleagues (2004b), the first documented use of a helmet in a football game occurred in 1893. The first football helmets were made of leather only. The use of helmets in football did not become mandatory in the NCAA until 1939; the NFL mandated the use of helmets in 1940. The first safety standards for football helmets did not appear until 1973.

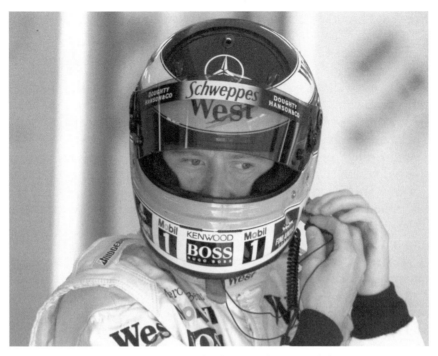

FIGURE 6.2   A helmet is a key piece of safety gear for automobile racers.
© Empics.

Most football helmets consist of a polycarbonate shell (about 4 mm thick) lined either with padding, air cells, or a combination of the two. These protective liners are designed to compress and absorb impact forces because the force is distributed across the entire surface area of the helmet (Barth et al. 2001; Biokinetics & Associates 2000; Broshek et al. 2004). Football helmets are subject to a recertification process in the United States to comply with prescribed standards. One major football manufacturer refuses to recertify any helmet over 10 years old (Powell and Dompier 2004).

Riddell, a maker of football helmets, introduced the "Revolution" helmet in 2002. The helmet was modified structurally to increase protection in the area of the mandibles (jaw) in an attempt to minimize impact forces to the head and thus decrease the likelihood of sustaining a concussion (for details of other modifications, go to www.riddell.com). The interim results of an ongoing study by Collins (2004) suggested a trend toward better protection (fewer concussive symptoms and quicker return to play) with the Revolution helmet. In 2004, Schutt (a football helmet manufacturer) introduced the "DNA" helmet. Promotional materials indicated an "advanced shell design," "smarter than foam padding/cushioning components," and a two-part air liner system (see www.SchuttDNA.com).

Interestingly, the CIS Group (2002) wrote, "For sports such as soccer, Australian football, and rugby, no sport-specific helmets have been shown to be of proven benefit in reducing rates of head injury" (p. 156). We are not aware of any current studies of possible hockey-helmet modification. Many hockey players now wear face visors for eye protection, yet many don't fasten their chinstraps tightly, which can diminish the protective power of the helmet. Broshek and associates (2004) provide an excellent discussion of the use of helmets in equestrian sports. Of note, they quote two surveys showing that the unattractive physical appearance of helmets was a major factor in nonuse among these athletes.

Helmets in various sports are now being equipped with a device (triaxial accelerometer) that is capable of measuring head acceleration and motion in high-speed crashes. Dr. Stephen Olvey and associates (2004) recently detailed the conceptualization, design, and implementation of this system in professional racing. Dr. Stefan Duma of Virginia Tech has piloted a similar effort in collegiate football (Duma et al. 2005).

The use of mouthguards appears to be routine in professional football and boxing but rather inconsistent in professional hockey. The same can be said for collegiate ice hockey. Kristen Hawn, ATC, and collaborators (2002) surveyed 127 NCAA-affiliated men's ice hockey programs and found that only 63% of athletes consistently wore mouthguards during competition. The CIS Group (2002), in discussing concussion prevention and mouthguards, concluded,

> Undoubtedly the use of correctly fitting mouthguards can reduce the rate of dental, orofacial [around the mouth and face], and mandibular [jaw] injuries. The evidence that they reduce cerebral injuries is largely theoretical, and the limited clinical evidence for a beneficial effect in reducing concussion rates has not been prospectively tested. (p. 156)

In other words, although mouthguards can prevent injuries to the face and teeth, there is no strong scientific evidence that they provide protection against concussion. McCrory (2001a) and Winters (2001) discuss mouthguard use more completely.

It should be noted that one study (Benson et al. 2002) showed that wearing a full face shield in collegiate ice hockey reduced the amount of time lost to concussion by over 50% compared with half-face shields. The Centers for Disease Control and Prevention published a pamphlet titled *Heads Up: Facts for Physicians About Mild Traumatic Brain Injuries* (undated). The CDC has recommended that helmets be worn while riding a motorcycle, bicycle, snowmobile, or all-terrain vehicle; when using a skateboard or in-line skates; during equestrian sports, snowboarding, and skiing; and while playing football, ice hockey, baseball, lacrosse, and softball.

The use of helmets in soccer has received a great deal of attention lately. The pros and cons have been addressed in the press and in the literature. In short, some believe that the use of helmets will provide a measure of protection against concussion, while others believe that the use of helmets might lead athletes to be more aggressive, thus leading to more injuries. A recent laboratory study by Steven Broglio, ATC, and associates (2003) evaluated the effectiveness of three headbands (circular bands made of an elastic, hard rubber material that cover the forehead and circumference of the cranium) in reducing peak impact force. Although all three headbands were effective to varying degrees, the authors commented, "The clinical effectiveness of these products remains to be seen" (p. 224). We look forward to the results of scientific studies that address the issue of whether helmets in soccer (or rugby or lacrosse) reduce concussive injury.

We know for sure that no helmet is concussion proof. We look forward to the results of scientific studies in progress assessing the newer helmets designed to decrease the potential for and severity of concussion. In the interim, we encourage athletes to wear well-fitted helmets, notify equipment managers of any worn or inadequate protective padding, tighten chin straps, and wear appropriately fitted mouthguards.

What Can We Do About Concussion?

First, let's take it seriously. The days of a concussion being dismissed as a simple "ding" or "a bell ringer" are over. We know many people (including athletes) who are more upset about dropping their laptop, cell phone, or PDA than receiving a hit to their own head. Again, you can buy a new computer or PDA, but you only get one brain.

Most of us are aware of the effects of concussion on the careers of many professional athletes. Keep in mind, however, that these are the high-profile athletes, the ones we hear about all the time. We don't read as frequently about the amateur, collegiate, or high school athletes who have to stop competing because of the effects of concussion. Maybe it's time to rethink our attitudes toward concussion, especially in younger athletes. Most players will play hurt. This action is not wise after a concussion because the player's concentration is off (and thus she is less attentive to the game). Eye–hand coordination is slowed, so stick or ball handling or pass catching is slower. Memory can be impaired, so a player may not remember which play was called or what his role in the play is supposed to be. Speed of information processing is off, so reaction times are slowed and the player may not make a pass or an adjustment quickly enough. This situation is not a recipe for success on the field.

Encourage players to use good padding in their helmets, tighten chinstraps, and wear mouthguards and face shields, as appropriate. Encourage them to report symptoms honestly and in a timely fashion. Although concussion should be taken seriously, it is not necessary to take on a gloom-and-doom attitude. Complete recovery is the typical outcome more than 90% of the time.

Make an attempt not to pressure a player about reporting clinical symptoms or performance on the neuropsychological tests, as anxiety can affect test performance and symptom reporting adversely. It would be silly to say that a player failed the neuropsychological tests, just as we wouldn't say that a player with a torn ACL (anterior cruciate ligament) failed the MRI. Do not pressure a player to minimize symptoms or return to play too quickly. The goal is to ensure safety and complete recovery before returning an athlete to play, which is the plain, simple truth *and* the smart thing to do.

New Research and the Future

While we've provided answers to many questions about concussion, we've almost certainly raised more questions. At times it may appear that the complexities of concussion are unsolvable, but we are optimistic and await future research for those answers.

New studies using advanced imaging techniques such as functional MRI (fMRI) may help us to learn more about the pathology of concussion, how it occurs, and the specific parts of the brain affected by it. Neuropsychology has already given us clues to this, and advancements in neuropsychological testing, especially as used in conjunction with fMRI, will tell us a great deal more. For example, the University of Pittsburgh's Sports Concussion Program has a grant from the National Institute of Health to study the relationship between neuropsychological test results and fMRI data in concussed athletes. Dr. Karen Johnston and colleagues at McGill University have been conducting similar studies. An example of their work is depicted in figure 6.3.

So many questions remain unanswered. For example, which symptoms in concussion are most important in predicting outcome? Is it safe to return an athlete to play if she has been asymptomatic for 15 minutes after a concussion? How many concussions are too many? Are these parameters the same for athletes at all levels of competition? Are there age and gender differences? Is there a genetic predisposition for one person to suffer a concussion more easily than another? Do genetics play a role in recovery times? Are genetics relevant to the issue of completeness of recovery postconcussion? Are there different patterns of healing based on these factors? We used to view loss of consciousness as most crucial, but now we know that this is not true. No doubt there will be many other surprises, and we anticipate the results of ongoing research to shed light on these issues.

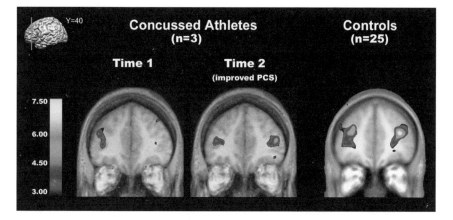

FIGURE 6.3 Composite fMRI data of concussed athletes with protracted postconcussion syndrome. The image on the right depicts normal brain activation in nonconcussed athletes, while the image on the left reflects diminished activation in concussed athletes shortly after a concussion. The middle image depicts intermediate activation during the recovery phase. PCS = postconcussion symptoms.

Courtesy of Karen Johnston, MD, PhD, Alain Ptito, PhD, and Jen-Kai Chen.

We hope that with advances in diagnostic techniques, new treatments will be developed both to maximize brain healing and to optimize a player's career. The search for evidence that concussions may or may not lead to long-term problems will unfold as scientifically sound, prospective, longitudinal studies are undertaken and completed in all high-risk sports and at various levels of competition.

Research Digest

The multistage procedure used to screen for dementia in the study by Plassman et al. (2000) included (sequentially) telephone screening; clinical, medical, and psychiatric histories; medication usage; family history of dementia; physical and neurological examination; neuropsychological testing; and ApoE genotyping. There were 548 veterans with head injury and 1,228 without head injury who completed all aspects of the study. The criteria for inclusion as a head-injured subject were documented head trauma in the military record occurring during military service; evidence of LOC, posttraumatic amnesia, and skull fracture; no penetration of the dura matter of the brain; and no marked cognitive impairment or neurological aftereffects 3 months after the injury.

The estimated risk for AD was estimated using a statistical model called proportional hazards. Mild head injury was defined as LOC or posttraumatic amnesia of less than 30 minutes, with no skull fracture. Moderate head injury was defined as LOC or posttraumatic amnesia of more than 30 minutes but less than 24 hours, and/or a skull fracture. Severe head injury was defined as LOC or posttraumatic amnesia for more than 24 hours.

Having any type of head injury increased a veteran's odds of developing dementia or AD by a factor of 2.23. Moderate head injury increased the risk for AD by a factor of 2.32, and severe head injury increased the risk for AD by a factor of 4.51. The authors also assessed whether the head-injured veterans had other military or nonmilitary head injuries (noted in the medical record or ascertained during the extensive interviews). The results were unchanged for all three groups, indicating that multiple head injuries did not change the risk outcome.

The ApoE genotyping results revealed no interaction effect between head injury and ApoE status on the risk of AD. These findings were in stark contrast to those reported by Jordan and colleagues (1997) in their study of boxers.

The Guo et al. (2000) study is known as the MIRAGE Study (Multi-Institutional Research in Alzheimer Genetic Epidemiology). This project was a collaborative effort assessing 2,233 patients with AD and 14,668 first-degree relatives at 13 centers in the United States, Canada, and Germany. A primary purpose was to assess the relationship between head injury and the development of AD. Head injury was assessed in this study as a "present" or "absent" variable (as opposed to mild, moderate, or severe, as was done in the Plassman study) by interviewing multiple informants and reviewing medical records.

The Sundstrom et al. study (2004) is a population-based, longitudinal study about aging among 3,500 adults in Sweden. Nine neuropsychological tests were administered to all participants at baseline; ApoE genotyping also was completed. Thirty-four adults were identified as having experienced a mild TBI after baseline testing had occurred. Eleven of the 34 adults were ApoE e4 positive. The authors reported that the ApoE e4-positive adults had a significantly decreased postinjury performance on three of the neuropsychological tests; such was not the case with the mild head-injured adults who were ApoE e4 negative.

Collins et al. (2002) studied 173 high school athletes who participated in the Sports Medicine Concussion Program at the University of Pittsburgh Medical Center. Complete concussion histories and preinjury (baseline) neuropsychological tests (ImPACT) were available on all players. Of the athletes studies, 34.7% of the players had never had a concussion, 33.5% had experienced one concussion, 15.6% had three concussions, 4.0% had four concussions, 1.2% had five concussions, and 2.3% reported having had six to nine concussions. These were high school athletes (more than 80% male) from Pennsylvania, Michigan, Illinois, Oregon, and Maine. Average age was about 16 years old. The athletes participated in the sports of football, soccer, basketball, hockey, lacrosse, volleyball, and wrestling. A formal-odds ratio (Collins et al. 2002) revealed that players with a history of three or more concussions were 9.3 times more likely than athletes with no prior concussion history to display three of the four on-field markers of concussion severity.

Iverson et al. (2004a) studied 19 amateur athletes from the Sports Concussion Program at the University of Pittsburgh Medical Center who had experienced three or more concussions. Eleven of the 19 were high school athletes; the remaining 8 athletes were collegiate. These athletes were then carefully matched with a group of 19 athletes with no prior history of concussion on the basis of age, education, participation level (high school or college), gender, sport, and days tested postinjury. Athletes of both groups had sustained a concussion during the current season. The average age of the athletes was about 18 years; over 90% were male, with average years of education being about 12. The majority was football players. Preinjury cognitive baseline data (ImPACT) was available for all athletes. On average, players were tested 1.7 days after the concussion. Iverson's group assessed ImPACT scores, on-field markers of concussion, and players' report of symptoms.

The NCAA Concussion studies (Guskiewicz et al. 2004) showed a positive correlation between reported number of previous concussions and the likelihood of having a concussion during the 3-year study. Players reporting a history of three or more prior concussions were three times more likely to have a concussion during the study than those players with no prior concussion history. The most frequently reported symptom was headache (85.2%), and the average amount of time required for symptom resolution was 82 hours (3.42 days).

Also of interest was the fact that among the 12 players who suffered another within-season concussion, 11 of the 12 concussions (91.7%) occurred within 10 days of the first concussion. This finding highlights the importance of allowing time for complete recovery from an initial concussion before exposing an athlete to the risk of another.

Essential Information for Athletes, Parents, and Coaches

This appendix provides a brief summary of the previous chapters, primarily designed to provide an overview of sport concussion for coaches, athletes, and family members. Clinicians can use this appendix as a useful communication tool when working with these individuals.

A concussion is an alteration in mental status or brain functioning resulting from a direct or indirect blow to the head. A person does not have to lose consciousness in order to sustain a concussion. Most sport concussions are mild and cause a transient disruption of the brain's normal electrical and chemical processes, leading to various signs and symptoms. Structural injury to the brain is relatively rare in sport concussion, but it can occur. Approximately 822 sport-related concussions occur in the United States every day. Your family doctor and the team athletic trainer are key players in the evaluation and treatment of sport concussion. A neuropsychologist may also be consulted to assess the effects of concussion on brain functioning; she will administer a battery of paper-and-pencil or computer-based tests to evaluate the cognitive effects of the concussion. The athletic trainer may also test balance (postural stability) because balance can be affected adversely after a concussion.

neurotransmitter—A naturally occurring substance in the brain that serves as a chemical messenger from one nerve cell to the next. Neurotransmitters allow neurons to communicate and serve as the biological basis for cognitive functioning.

During a concussion the brain undergoes a series of chemical events and changes that can last for a week or even longer. These chemical changes involve alterations in numerous substances, including calcium, potassium, and **neurotransmitters** in the brain. Blood flow to the brain also tends to be reduced after a concussion. In most cases, the brain heals the chemical and blood-flow abnormalities on its own. The U.S. Food and Drug Administration has not approved any medications for the treatment of concussion, and at present there is no proven way to speed up the process of healing the brain after a concussion. Rest, avoiding exertion (physical and mental exertion can worsen the symptoms of a concussion), and the prevention of a premature return to play (which can cause the athlete to run the risk of incurring another concussion) are the only known effective treatment strategies.

Concussion in sport has become a major problem. Disability and death have occurred as a result of concussive head injuries, especially at the high school level. Second-impact syndrome (SIS) is a condition that occurs when an athlete who sustains an initial head injury (usually a concussion) experiences a second head injury before symptoms associated with the first injury have cleared. Although quite rare, SIS can be life threatening for young athletes. It is important to realize, however, that although the rate of concussion incidents in sport has grown, in the United States an adolescent has a greater chance of being killed while riding a bicycle than while playing organized sports.

Awareness of sport concussion peaked in the United States at the turn of the 21st century. It is now a commonly discussed topic in the media and in professional journals and textbooks. According to published data, the odds of a contact sport athlete sustaining a concussion while playing organized sports are roughly 5% per season. This percentage may be an underestimation, however, given that athletes often fail to recognize symptoms or report concussions to trainers or doctors.

Signs and Symptoms

Some of the immediate signs that an athlete has sustained a concussion include the following:

- Appears dazed
- Is confused about the play, score, or opponent
- Exhibits decreased playing ability
- Displays poor balance, lack of coordination
- Answers questions slowly
- Exhibits personality or behavioral changes
- Is unaware of time, date, and place
- Runs in the wrong direction
- Has a vacant stare; looks glassy eyed
- Forgets plays or events that occurred before the impact (retrograde amnesia)
- Forgets plays or events that occurred after the impact (anterograde amnesia)
- Loses consciousness
- Experiences a seizure (rare)

Some of the more common symptoms of concussion include the following:

- Headache
- Nausea and vomiting
- Balance problems
- Double or blurred vision
- Sensitivity to light (photosensitivity)
- Sensitivity to noise (phonosensitivity)
- Feeling sluggish, "foggy," or "just not right"
- Feeling "dinged" or "dazed," having "bell rung"
- Seeing stars or flashing lights
- Ringing in the ears
- Changes in sleep patterns
- Poor concentration

- Memory problems
- Drowsiness
- Low energy, feeling slowed down
- Irritability
- Sadness
- Anxiety and nervousness
- More emotional than usual
- Feeling "pressure in the head"

These symptoms are usually self-limiting and clear up within a week.

Assessment, Evaluation, and Treatment

The clinical assessment of concussion can be performed on the sideline with mental-status questions and structured cognitive tests. Examples of mental-status questions for the assessment of sport-related concussion include asking the athlete the score of the game, which quarter or period it is, and who won the previous game. Neuropsychological testing is a more thorough strategy in the evaluation of the cognitive symptoms of concussion. These are paper-and-pencil or computer-based tests that measure brain functions such as memory, concentration, and speed of information processing. Neuropsychological testing and other sideline mental-status tests are most useful when a preseason baseline score on the test has been obtained on each athlete. The athlete's postconcussion test scores, in tandem with an assessment of clinical signs and symptoms, can then be compared with baseline scores to assess the severity of the concussion and to monitor recovery. Cost- and time-effective baseline neuropsychological testing is now available through sports neuropsychologists; we strongly urge parents of contact- and collision-sport athletes to have their children undergo baseline neuropsychological testing.

Structural **neuroimaging** (brain) scans, such as **computed axial tomography (CT)** or **magnetic resonance imaging (MRI)**, are not always required after sport-related concussion. In fact, these tests are found to be normal more than 90% of the time after mild sport concussions. The presence of specific neurological signs (detected by a physician, athletic trainer, or nurse) or the prolonged presence of postconcussion symptoms would warrant the consideration of a

CT or MRI of the brain. Newer functional brain-imaging technologies (such as positron emission tomography [PET] scans and functional MRI [fMRI]) measure oxygen, glucose, and blood-flow patterns in the brain and show a great deal of promise for the future. Balance testing may be a useful adjunctive strategy in assessing the postural-stability effects of concussion.

More than 25 grading scales for concussion have been published, and two in particular are used commonly to assess sport concussion. Most of these scales were not derived from scientific study but have been based on expert and consensus opinion. The true values of a grading scale are in its ability to accurately classify concussion severity and to predict recovery and outcome. No grading scale has yet to meet these criteria from a scientific viewpoint. The Concussion in Sport (CIS) Group (2002) did not endorse any particular grading scale and emphasized the need for each concussion to be assessed and treated individually.

Since the late-1990s, structured programs for the evaluation and assessment of concussion have occurred in the NFL, NHL, and NCAA. Greater effort has been made at all levels of competition to increase awareness of concussion and to better evaluate and treat this common brain injury. Professional organizations have also been busy delineating guidelines for the assessment and management of concussion in athletes. Neurologists, neurosurgeons, orthopedic surgeons, and multidisciplinary groups have published concussion guidelines. The Concussion in Sport Group (CIS), an international group of sport concussion experts, has presented the most recent guidelines (2002, 2005). We consider these guidelines to be the gold standard for concussion assessment and management.

The CIS guidelines emphasize a multistep rehabilitation program under the direction of a qualified professional. The first step postconcussion is complete rest until all symptoms resolve. If baseline neuropsychological testing has been done, the test scores should have returned to the athlete's baseline. If neuroimaging has been performed, the results should be normal. The next step

neuroimaging—The application of various types of X-ray and nuclear methods to produce radiographs (images) of the central nervous system. Computed tomography (CT) and magnetic resonance imaging (MRI) are the most common neuroimaging methods.

computed axial tomography (CAT, or CT)—A specialized X-ray technique that allows visualization of detailed areas of the body in a specific plane.

magnetic resonance imaging (MRI)—A specialized diagnostic technique that utilizes magnetic, X-ray, and nuclear methods to provide a detailed image of specific body areas.

after symptom resolution is light aerobic activity such as walking or stationary cycling. Sport-specific training follows and might include running in soccer or skating in hockey. The next step is noncontact training drills, followed by full-contact training (after medical clearance, including a normal neurological exam). Return to game play is the final step. The CIS group emphasized that each step in the rehabilitation program may take a day to complete and that the recurrence of symptoms at any point necessitates stepping back to the prior level of rehabilitation.

At present, there are no medications approved in the United States (or anywhere else in the world) specifically for concussion. Some doctors are using various medications for the treatment of specific, prolonged concussion symptoms (for example, migraine-type headache), and the off-label use of various drugs has been noted in many (nonsport-related) concussive injuries. Rest (and the prevention of another concussion) is the primary treatment at present. The athlete should not engage in exertional activities (physical or mental) before beginning the structured and supervised rehabilitation program because these activities can worsen the symptoms of concussion and prolong the rehabilitation period. It is important to recognize (as Dr. Mark Lovell has said), that the brain is not a muscle; exercise will not help an athlete recover from a concussion initially. Design changes have been made by football-helmet manufacturers in an attempt to improve protection against concussion. A concussion-proof helmet, however, does not yet exist.

Sport-Specific Concerns

arachnoid cyst—A closed cavity or sac containing a liquid or semisolid material found in the spiderlike covering between the brain and the skull.

subdural hematoma—A localized collection of blood (and spinal fluid) in the space underneath the outer covering of the brain (the dura) usually resulting from a laceration in the brain and/or a tear in a blood vessel.

Although clear evidence proves that concussions occur in soccer and that brain function can be affected adversely by them, there is no convincing evidence to indicate that heading the ball in soccer causes cognitive deficits in the vast majority of athletes. Soccer athletes with **arachnoid cysts** of the brain may be at greater risk for the development of a **subdural hematoma** after repeated heading of the ball or concussion.

Boxing is the only sport where one of the stated purposes is to inflict a concussion on one's opponent. Available studies suggest a significant risk for cognitive difficulties later in life for professional boxers who have prolonged careers. A specific genetic risk factor (the Apolipoprotein E4 allele, or ApoE e4) has been proposed. Less convincing evidence for significant long-term cognitive impairment has been reported in amateur boxers. Limiting one's exposure to boxing is perhaps the safest alternative.

The risk for concussion in cycling is evident; more cycling deaths occur in the United States annually than in any other recreational sport. Everyone should wear a helmet while cycling. The same can be said for equestrian sports, although studies indicate that some equestrian athletes do not wear helmets due to cosmetic (personal appearance) reasons (Broshek et al. 2004).

The introduction of better-designed football helmets may offer athletes improved protection against the effects of concussion; we eagerly await the results of studies in progress designed to test this possibility. We await further studies of the role of ApoE e4 in short- and long-term studies of sport concussion. A preliminary study, which reported on professional football athletes (Kutner et al. 2000), suggested that older athletes who were positive for the ApoE e4 allele had lower cognitive test scores and merits further formal investigation. It should be emphasized that at the present time there is no scientific evidence to support a specific magic number of concussions that would mandate retirement or cessation of competition.

We are not aware of any current attempts to modify helmets in professional hockey but believe that the severity of concussions experienced in hockey could be truncated (at least in part) with better padding and improved helmet design. Regular helmet inspection and replacement of worn parts, along with appropriate enforcement of the rules for wearing helmets (that is, tightened chinstraps), could also result in lessened effects of concussion.

Long-Term Effects

No answer has yet been found to the question of how many concussions are too many. Preliminary studies have linked concussion to an increased risk of Alzheimer's disease and major depression in the *general population*. A survey study of retired NFL athletes has not shown a strong relationship between concussion and Alzheimer's disease but did indicate a higher incidence of major depression later in life in athletes who experienced multiple concussions. Preliminary studies (Collins et al. 2002; Iverson et al. 2004a) are suggesting that the effects of multiple concussions may be cumulative in high school and collegiate athletes, evidenced by worse on-the-field indicators of concussion (for example, confusion, disorientation, amnesia), worse scores on neuropsychological tests, and a protracted resolution of concussion symptoms.

Return to Play

Consideration of all aspects of the game and its risks should be considered when deciding whether an athlete should return to play. If it is decided that the athlete will return to play, it is recommended that every athlete follow the guidelines outlined in the CIS Group's (2002, 2005) documents to maximize safety. This includes completing a preseason concussion-symptom checklist, taking baseline sport-concussion neuropsychological tests, and having routine medical examinations. In the end, return to play is a medical decision that should not be made by a parent or an athlete. Each case is handled individually, but in general, an athlete should not be returned to play until all symptoms have cleared, both at rest and with exertion. If done, neuropsychological test scores should have returned to baseline. Finally, the athlete should have completed a graduated, sport-specific rehabilitation program under the supervision of an athletic trainer and physician.

Educating Athletes About Concussion

First and foremost, we hope that this book fills a needed information gap for physicians, athletic trainers, psychologists, coaches, therapists, and other sports professionals in the understanding of concussion. Surprisingly, few formal programs are available to educate athletes about concussions. For example, Dr. Kevin Kaut and colleagues (2003) surveyed collegiate athletes during the 1995 to 2001 athletic seasons. The results indicated that nearly one-third of the athletes had sustained a blow to the head causing dizziness (or other physical symptoms). Less than 20% of the athletes were aware that these symptoms represented a probable concussion, and over half continued to play despite the presence of these symptoms. More than half of the athletes were deemed as having knowledge deficits about concussion.

These results in *collegiate* athletes mirror McCrea's findings of underreported concussions in nearly half of *high school* football players (2004). Delaney and colleagues (2000) found that 80% of *professional* football players were unaware that they had sustained a concussion despite being symptomatic. Taken together, these studies are worrisome and indicate a lack of awareness about concussion symptoms and consequences among athletes at all levels of competition. We believe the time has come to include concussion education, including symptom recognition and appropriate medical management, for all athletes. Sports medicine professionals are in an excellent position to take the lead in this endeavor. In its Position Statement on sport-related concussion, the National Athletic Trainers' Association (NATA) called for athletic trainers to play an active role in educating athletes, coaches, and parents about concussion and the potential risks of playing while still symptomatic (Guskiewicz et al. 2004).

Doctors Janet Jankowiak and Elizabeth Roaf (2004), writing in the "Patient Page" section of the journal *Neurology,* present a brief but concise educational overview of sport concussion for athletes and their parents, coaches, and medical personnel. At the professional sports level, the National Hockey League Players Association has developed an educational video (addressing the roles of helmets and padding, chinstraps, visors, mouthguards, and playing "heads up") that is shown to all players during training camp. This video was first introduced to all NHL teams during training camp in the 2002-2003 season. It is a sensible, factual documentary hosted by Brett Lindros (an ex-NHL player whose career was cut short by concussions) that emphasizes prevention. We are not aware of any formal directives by the NFL or NCAA regarding player education about concussion. What we have observed in the NHL and NFL is an informal mentoring process whereby athletes who have dealt with concussions provide information to their peers who are now dealing with the problem. The grassroots approach is a powerful one.

Neurosurgeons and neuroscience nurses across Canada and the United States began the ThinkFirst Foundation, an organization devoted to the prevention of traumatic injuries in children. Safety education is a primary focus, and many of ThinkFirst's programs are geared toward young athletes. For more information, go to www.thinkfirst.ca. The Pashby Sports Safety Fund of Canada previously had a Web site specific to hockey and concussion, but it has been merged with the ThinkFirst Web site. A number of other educational tools and resources for the community are available and are listed in appendix B.

appendix b

Resources

Computer-Based Neuropsychological Testing for Sport Concussion

CogSport www.cogsport.com (now known as "Concussion Sentinel")

HeadMinder www.headminder.com

Immediate Postconcussion Assessment and Cognitive Testing (ImPACT) www.impacttest.com

Sideline-Assessment Strategies

McGill Abbreviated Concussion Evaluation. For ordering information, contact Dr. Karen Johnston at karen.johnston@staff.mcgill.ca.

SideLine ImPACT. For ordering information, contact Labiba Russo at lrusso@impacttest.com, or go to www.impacttest.com.

Sport Concussion Assessment Tool (SCAT). Published in the 2005 issues of the *Clinical Journal of Sport Medicine, British Journal of Sports Medicine,* and *The Physician and Sportsmedicine.*

Standardized Assessment of Concussion (Second Edition). For ordering information, contact senior author Dr. Michael McCrea at michael.mccrea@phci.com, or call 1-800-326-2011, extension 2156.

General Resources for Sport Concussion

American Academy of Neurology www.aan.com

Brain Injury Association of America www.biausa.org

Canadian Academy of Sport Medicine (CASM) www.casm-acms.org

Centers for Disease Control www.cdc.gov/ncipc/tbi

Concussion in Sport (CIS) Group (2001) and (2004) Consensus Statements http://bjsm.bmjjournals.com/searchall/ (use keywords "concussion Vienna")

Institute of Medicine Conference, 2002: Is Soccer Bad for Children's Health? http://books.nap.edu (search for "0309083443")

International Olympic Committee www.olympic.org

National Academy of Neuropsychology www.nanonline.org

National Athletic Trainer's Association www.nata.org

National Athletic Trainer's Association Position Statement on Management of Sport-Related Concussion www.nata.org (click on "Public Information," then "NATA Statements")

National Bicycle Safety Network www.cdc.gov/ncipc/bike

National Collegiate Athletic Association (NCAA) www.ncaa.org

National Football League (NFL) www.nfl.com

National Hockey League (NHL) www.nhl.com

ThinkFirst Foundation www.thinkfirst.ca

United States Olympic Committee (USOC) www.olympic-usa.org

References

Abreau F, Templer DI, Schuyler BA, et al. Neuropsychological assessment of soccer players. *Neuropsychology*, 1990, *4*, 175-181.

American Academy of Neurology Report of the Quality Standards Committee. Practice parameter: The management of concussion in sports (summary statement). *Neurology*, 1997, *48*, 581-585.

American Congress of Rehabilitative Medicine. Report of the Mild Traumatic Brain Injury Committee of the Head Injury Interdisciplinary Special Interest Group: Definition of mild traumatic brain injury. *Journal of Head Trauma Rehabilitation*, 1993, *8*, 86-87.

American Psychiatric Association. *Diagnostic and statistical manual of mental disorders* (4th ed.). Washington, D.C.: American Psychiatric Association, 1994.

Apuzzo, MLJ. Carpe diem: Sports neurosurgery. *Neurosurgery*, 2003, *52*, 1-2.

Asplund CA, McKeag DB, Olsen CH. Sport-related concussion: Factors associated with prolonged return to play. *Clinical Journal of Sport Medicine*, 2004, *14*, 339-343.

Bailes JE. *Boxing/martial arts and concussion*. Paper presented at the New Developments in Sports-Related Concussion Conference, Pittsburgh, July 2004.

Bailes JE, Cantu RC. Head injury in athletes. *Neurosurgery*, 2001, *48*, 26-45.

Bailes JE, Guskiewicz K, Marshall S. Recurrent sport-related concussion linked to clinical depression. Paper presented at the 71st Annual Meeting of the American Association of Neurological Surgeons, San Diego, April, 2003.

Bailes JE, Lovell MR, Maroon JC. *Sports-related concussion*. St. Louis: Quality Medical Publishing, 1999.

Barnes BC, Cooper L, Kirkendall DT, et al. Concussion history in elite male and female soccer players. *American Journal of Sports Medicine*, 1998, *26*, 433-438.

Barr WB, McCrea M. Sensitivity and specificity of standardized neurocognitive testing immediately following sports concussion. *Journal of the International Neuropsychological Society*, 2001, *7*, 693-702.

Barth JT, Alves WM, Ryan TV, et al. Mild head injury in sports: Neuropsychological sequelae and recovery of function. In Levin HS, Eisenberg HM, Benton AL, et al. (Eds.), *Mild head injury* (pp. 257-275). New York: Oxford Press, 1989.

Barth JT, Freeman JR, Broshek DK, et al. Acceleration-deceleration sports-related concussion: The gravity of it all. *Journal of Athletic Training*, 2001, *36*, 253-256.

Bazarian J. *Blood serum markers of brain injury.* Paper presented at the New Developments in Sports-Related Concussion Conference, Pittsburgh, July 2004.

Bender SD, Barth JT, Irby J. *Historical perspectives.* In Lovell MR, Echemendia RJ, Barth JT, Collins MW (Eds.), *Traumatic brain injury in sports: An international neuropsychological perspective.* Lisse, The Netherlands: Swets & Zeitlinger, 2004.

Benson BW, Rose MS, Meeuwisse WH. The impact of face shield use on concussion in ice hockey: A multivariate analysis. *British Journal of Sport Medicine,* 2002, *36,* 27-32.

Biokinetics & Associates. Equestrian headgear standards. *American Medical Equestrian Association News,* 2000, *11,* 1-3.

Bleiberg J, Cernich AN, Cameron K, et al. Duration of cognitive impairment after sports concussion. *Neurosurgery,* 2004, *54,* 1073-1080.

Bloom GA, Horton AS, McCrory P, et al. Sport psychology and concussion: New impacts to explore. *British Journal of Sports Medicine,* 2004, *38,* 519-521.

Boden BP, Kirkendall DT, Garrett WE, Jr. Concussion incidence in elite college soccer players. *American Journal of Sports Medicine,* 1998, *26,* 238-241.

Broglio SP, Guskiewicz KM, Sell TC, et al. No acute changes in postural control after soccer heading. *British Journal of Sports Medicine,* 2004, *38,* 561-567.

Broglio SP, Yan-Ying J, Broglio MD, et al. The efficacy of soccer headgear. *Journal of Athletic Training,* 2003, *38,* 220-224.

Brooks J. *Gender issues in brain injury.* In Lovell MR, Echemendia RJ, Barth JT, et al. (Eds.), *Traumatic brain injury in sports: An international neuropsychological perspective.* Lisse, The Netherlands: Swets & Zeitlinger, 2004.

Broshek DK, Brazil AM, Freeman JR, Barth, JT. *Equestrian sports.* In Lovell MR, Echemendia RJ, Barth JT, et al. (Eds.), *Traumatic brain injury in sports: An international neuropsychological perspective.* Lisse, The Netherlands: Swets & Zeitlinger, 2004.

Bruce JM, Echemendia RJ. Concussion history predicts self-reported symptoms before and following a concussive event. *Neurology,* 2004, *63,* 1516-1518.

Burke CJ. *Update from the National Hockey League (NHL).* Paper presented at the New Developments in Sports-Related Concussion Conference, Pittsburgh, July, 2002.

Burke CJ. *Update from the National Hockey League.* Paper presented at the New Developments in Sport-Related Concussion Conference, Pittsburgh, July 2004.

Canadian Academy of Sport Medicine Concussion Committee. Guidelines for assessment and management of sport-related concussion. *Clinical Journal of Sport Medicine,* 2000, *10,* 209-211.

Cantu RC. Guidelines for return to contact sports after a cerebral concussion. *The Physician and Sportsmedicine,* 1986, *14,* 75-83.

Cantu RC. Posttraumatic retrograde and anterograde amnesia: Pathophysiology and implications in grading and safe return to play. *Journal of Athletic Training,* 2001, *36,* 244-248.

Cantu RC. Athletic head injury. *Current Sports Medicine Reports*, 2003, *2*, 117-119.

Cantu RC. Sport: Challenge and opportunity. *Neurosurgery*, 2003, *52*, 2-3.

Cantu RC, Mueller FO. Brain injury-related fatalities in American football, 1945-1999. *Neurosurgery*, 2003, *52*, 846-853.

Cantu RC, Voy R. Second-impact syndrome: A risk in any contact sport. *The Physician and Sportsmedicine*, 1995, *23*, 27-34.

Carroll LJ, Cassidy JD, Holm L, et al. Methodological issues and research recommendations for mild traumatic brain injury: The WHO Collaborating Centre Task Force on Mild Traumatic Brain Injury. *Journal of Rehabilitative Medicine*, 2004, Supplement, *43*, 113-125.

Casson IR, Siegel O, Sham R, et al. Brain damage in modern boxers. *Journal of the American Medical Association*, 1984, *251*, 2663-2667.

Centers for Disease Control and Prevention. Sport-related recurrent brain injuries. *Morbidity and Mortality Weekly Report MMWR*, 1997, *46*, 224-227.

Centers for Disease Control. *Heads up: Facts for physicians about mild traumatic brain injury (MTBI)*. Department of Health and Human Services, undated.

Chen JK, Johnston KM, Frey S, et al. Functional abnormalities in symptomatic concussed athletes: An fMRI study. *NeuroImage*, 2004, *22*, 68-82.

Collie A, Maruff P, Makdissi M, et al. CogSport: Reliability and correlation with conventional cognitive tests used in postconcussion medical evaluations. *Clinical Journal of Sport Medicine*, 2003, *13*, 28-32.

Collins MW. *Computer-based neuropsychological testing*. Paper presented at the New Developments in Sports-Related Concussion conference, Pittsburgh, July 2004.

Collins MW, Field M, Lovell MR, et al. Relationship between post-concussion headache and neuropsychological test performance in high school athletes. *American Journal of Sports Medicine*, 2003a, *31*,168-173.

Collins MW, Grindel SH, Lovell MR, et al. Relationship between concussion and neuropsychological performance in college football players. *Journal of the American Medical Association*, 1999, *282*, 964-970.

Collins MW, Iverson GL, Lovell MR, et al. On-field predictors of neuropsychological and symptom deficit following sports-related concussion. *Clinical Journal of Sport Medicine*, 2003b, *13*, 222-229.

Collins MW, Lovell MR, Iverson GL, et al. Cumulative effects of concussion in high school athletes. *Neurosurgery*, 2002, *51*, 1175-1179.

Collins MW, Lovell MR, McKeag DB. Current issues in managing sports-related concussion. *Journal of the American Medical Association*, 1999, *282*, 2283-2285.

Concussion in Rodeo Group. Agreement statement from the 1st international rodeo research and clinical care conference. *Clinical Journal of Sport Medicine*, 2005, *15*, 192-195.

Concussion in Sport Group. Summary and agreement statement of the First International Symposium on Concussion in Sport, Vienna, 2001. *Clinical Journal of Sport Medicine*, 2002, *12*, 6-11.

Concussion in Sport Group. Summary and agreement statement of the Second International Symposium on Concussion in Sport, Prague, 2004. Published in the April 2005 issues of *The Physician and Sportsmedicine 33, Vol 4, British Journal of Sports Medicine 39,* 196-204, and the *Clinical Journal of Sport Medicine 15,* 48-55.

Congress of Neurological Surgeons: Proceedings of the Congress of Neurological Surgeons in 1964: Report of the Ad Hoc Committee to Study Head Injury Nomenclature. *Clinical Neurosurgery,* 1966, *12,* 386-394.

Covassin T, Swanik, CB, Sachs ML. Sex differences and the incidence of concussions among collegiate athletes. *Journal of Athletic Training,* 2003, *38,* 238-244.

Delaney JS. Head injuries presenting to emergency departments in the United States from 1990 to 1999 for ice hockey, soccer, and football. *Clinical Journal of Sport Medicine,* 2004, *14,* 80-87.

Delaney JS, Lacroix VJ, Gagne C, et al. Concussions among university football and soccer players: A pilot study. *Clinical Journal of Sport Medicine,* 2001, *11,* 234-240.

Delaney JS, Lacroix VJ, Leclerc S, et al. Concussion during the 1997 Canadian Football League season. *Clinical Journal of Sport Medicine,* 2000, *10,* 9-14.

Delaney JS, Lacroix VJ, Leclerc S, et al. Concussions among university football and soccer players. *Clinical Journal of Sport Medicine,* 2002, *12,* 331-338.

Demetriades AK, McEvoy AW, Kitchen ND. Subdural haematoma associated with an arachnoid cyst after repetitive minor heading injury in ball games. *British Journal of Sports Medicine,* 2004, *38,* e8.

Dick RW. A summary of head and neck injuries in collegiate athletics using the NCAA injury surveillance system. In Hoerner EF (Ed.), *Head and neck injuries in sports.* Philadelphia: American Society for Testing Materials, 1994.

Downs DS, Abwender D. Neuropsychological impairment in soccer athletes. *Journal of Sports Medicine and Physical Fitness,* 2002, *42,* 103-107.

Duma SM, Manoogian SJ, Bussone WR, et al. Analysis of real-time head accelerations in collegiate football players. *Clinical Journal of Sport Medicine,* 2005, *15,* 1-8.

Echemendia RJ. *Neuropsychological assessment of college athletes: The Penn State Concussion Program.* Paper presented at the annual meeting of the National Academy of Neuropsychology, Las Vegas, 1997.

Echemendia RJ, Cantu RC. Return to play following brain injury. In Lovell MR, Echemendia RJ, Barth JT, et al (Eds.), *Traumatic brain injury in sports: An international neuropsychological perspective.* Lisse, The Netherlands: Swets & Zeitlinger, 2004.

Echemendia RJ, Julian LJ. Mild traumatic brain injury in sports: Neuropsychology's contribution to a developing field. *Neuropsychology Review,* 2001, *11,* 69-88.

Echemendia RJ, Putukian M, Macklin RS, et al. Neuropsychological test performance prior to and following sports-related mild traumatic brain injury. *Clinical Journal of Sport Medicine,* 2001, *11,* 23-31.

Erlanger D, Kaushik T, Cantu R., et al. Symptom-based assessment of the severity of concussion. *Journal of Neurosurgery*, 2003, *98*, 477-484.

Erlanger DM, Kutner KC, Barth JT, et al. Neuropsychology of sports-related head injury: Dementia pugilistica to post concussion syndrome. *The Clinical Neuropsychologist*, 1999, *13*, 193-209.

Ferrara MS, McCrea M, Peterson CL, et al. A survey of practice patterns in concussion assessment and management. *Journal of Athletic Training*, 2001, *36*, 145-149.

Field M, Collins MW, Lovell MR, et al. Does age play a role in recovery from sports-related concussion? A comparison of high school and collegiate athletes. *Journal of Pediatrics*, 2003, *142*, 546-553.

Genin, G. Personal communication. November 2, 2004.

Giza CC, Hovda DA. The neurometabolic cascade of concussion. *Journal of Athletic Training*, 2001, *36*, 228-235.

Giza CC, Hovda DA. The pathophysiology of traumatic brain injury. In Lovell MR, Echemendia RJ, Barth JT, et al. (Eds.), *Traumatic brain injury in sports: An international neuropsychological perspective*. Lisse, The Netherlands: Swets & Zeitlinger, 2004.

Goodman D, Gaetz M, Meichenbaum D. Concussions in hockey: There is cause for concern. *Medicine and Science in Sports and Exercise,* 2001, *12*, 2004-2009.

Grindel SH. Epidemiology and pathophysiology of minor traumatic brain injury. *Current Sports Medicine Reports*, 2003, *2*, 18-23.

Grindel SH, Lovell MR, Collins MW. The assessment of sport-related concussion: The evidence behind neuropsychological testing and management. *Clinical Journal of Sport Medicine*, 2001, *11*, 134-143.

Guo Z, Cupples LA, Kurz A, et al. Head injury and the risk of AD in the MIRAGE study. *Neurology*, 2000, *54*, 1316-1323.

Guskiewicz KM. Postural stability assessment following concussion: One piece of the puzzle. *Clinical Journal of Sport Medicine*, 2001, *11*, 182-189.

Guskiewicz, KM. Assessment of postural stability following sports-related concussion. *Current Sports Medicine Reports*, 2003, *2*, 24-30.

Guskiewicz KM, Bruce SL, Cantu RC, et al. National Athletic Trainers' Association position statement: Management of sport-related concussion. *Journal of Athletic Training*, 2004, *39*, 280-297.

Guskiewicz KM, Marshall SW, Broglio SP, et al. No evidence of impaired neurocognitive performance in collegiate soccer players. *The American Journal of Sports Medicine*, 2002, *30*, 157-162.

Guskiewicz KM, McCrea M, Marshall SW, et al. Cumulative effects associated with recurrent concussion in collegiate football players: The NCAA concussion study. *Journal of the American Medical Association*, 2003, *290*, 2549-2555.

Guskiewicz KM, Weaver NL, Padua DA, et al. Epidemiology of concussion in collegiate and high school football players. *American Journal of Sports Medicine*, 2000, *28*, 643-650.

Haglund Y, Erikson E. Does amateur boxing lead to chronic brain damage? A review of some recent investigations. *American Journal of Sports Medicine,* 1993, *21,* 97-109.

Hawn KL, Visser MF, Sexton PJ. Enforcement of mouthguard use and athlete compliance in National Collegiate Athletic Association men's collegiate ice hockey competition. *Journal of Athletic Training,* 2002, *37,* 204-208.

Heck JF, Clarke KS, Peterson TR, et al. National Athletic Trainers' Association position statement: Head-down contact and spearing in tackle football. *Journal of Athletic Training,* 2004, *39,* 101-111.

Hinton-Bayre AD, Geffen GM. Contemporary classifications of concussion severity and short-term neuropsychological outcome. *British Journal of Sports Medicine,* 2002, *36,* 217.

Holsinger T, Steffens DC, Phillips C et al. Head injury in early adulthood and lifetime risk of depression. *Archives of General Psychiatry,* 2002, *59,* 17-24.

Hovda DA, Prins M, Becker DP, et al. Neurobiology of concussion. In Bailes JE, Lovell MR, Maroon, JC (Eds.), *Sports-related concussion* (pp. 12-51). St. Louis: Quality Medical Publishing, 1999.

Hurley RA, McGowan JC, Arfanakis K, et al. Traumatic axonal injury: Novel insights into evolution and identification. *Journal of Neuropsychiatry and Clinical Neuroscience,* 2004, *16,* 1-7.

Institute of Medicine. Is soccer bad for children's heads? Summary of the IOM workshop on neuropsychological consequences of head impact in youth soccer, 2002, Washington, D.C.: National Academy Press.

Iverson GL, Gaetz M, Lovell MR, et al. Cumulative effects of concussion in amateur athletes. *Brain Injury,* 2004a, *18,* 433-443.

Iverson GL, Gaetz M, Lovell MR, et al. Relation between subjective fogginess and neuropsychological testing following concussion. *Journal of the International Neuropsychological Society,* 2004b, *10,* 904-906.

Janda DH, Bir CA, Cheney AL. An evaluation of the cumulative concussive effects of soccer heading in the youth population. *Injury Control and Safety Promotion,* 2002, *9,* 25-31.

Jankowiak J, Roaf, E. "It's just a ding, Coach; I can play"—But should he? *Neurology,* 2004, *63,* E15.

Johnston KM. Hockey concussion reporting improved. *Canadian Journal of Neurological Sciences,* 2003, *30,* 183.

Johnston KM, Bloom GA, Ramsay J, et al. Current concepts in concussion rehabilitation. *Current Sports Medicine Reports,* 2004, *3,* 316-323.

Johnston KM, Chankowsky JC, Guerin M, et al. Neuroimaging in concussion. *Neuroimage Bulletin,* 2001a, *17,* 2-5.

Johnston KM, Lassonde M, Ptito A. A contemporary neurosurgical approach to sport-related head injury: The McGill concussion protocol. *Journal of the American College of Surgeons,* 2001a, *192,* 515-524.

Johnston KM, McCrory P, Mohtadi NG, et al. Evidence-based review of sport-related concussion: Clinical science. *Clinical Journal of Sport Medicine,* 2001b, *11,* 150-159.

Johnston KM, Ptito A, Chankowsky JC, et al. New frontiers in diagnostic imaging in concussive head injury. *Clinical Journal of Sport Medicine*, 2001c, *11*, 166-175.

Jordan SE, Green GA, Galanty HL, et al. Acute and chronic brain injury in United States National Team soccer players. *American Journal of Sports Medicine*, 1996, *24*, 205-210.

Jordan BD, Relkin NR, Ravdin LD, et al. Apolipoprotein E e4 associated with chronic traumatic brain injury in boxing. *Journal of the American Medical Association*, 1997, *278*, 136-140.

Kaut KP, DePompei R, Kerr J, et al. Reports of head injury and symptom knowledge among college athletes: Implications for assessment and educational intervention. *Clinical Journal of Sport Medicine*, 2003, *13*, 213-221.

Kelly JP. Traumatic brain injury and concussion in sports. *Journal of the American Medical Association*, 1999, *282*, 989-991.

Kelly JP. Loss of consciousness: Pathophysiology and implications in grading and safe return to play. *Journal of Athletic Training*, 2001, *36*, 249-252.

Kirkendall DT, Garrett WE. Heading in soccer: Integral skill or grounds for cognitive dysfunction? *Journal of Athletic Training*, 2001, *36*, 328-333.

Kirkendall DT, Jordan SE, Garrett WE. Heading and heading injuries in soccer. *Sports Medicine*, 2001, *31*, 369-386.

Koenig HG, George LK, Larson DB, et al. Depressive symptoms and nine-year survival of 1,001 male veterans hospitalized with medical illness. *American Journal of Geriatric Psychiatry*, 1999, *7*, 124-131.

Kontos A, Collins MW, Russo S. An introduction to sports concussion for the sport psychology consultant. *Journal of Applied Sport Psychology*, 2004, *16*, 220-235.

Koss R, Ohler K, Barolin, GS. Effect of heading in soccer on the head: A quantifying EEG study of soccer players (in German). *EEG EMG Z elektroenzephalogr. Elektromyogr. Verwandte Geb.*, 1983, *14*, 209-212.

Kutner KC, Erlanger DM, Tsai J, et al. Lower cognitive performance in older football players possessing apolipoprotein E e4. *Neurosurgery*, 2000, *47*, 651-657.

Leclerc S, Lassonde M, Delaney JS, et al. Recommendations for grading of concussion in athletes. *Sports Medicine*, 2001, *31*, 629-636.

Levy ML, Ozgur BM, Berry C, et al. Analysis and evolution of head injury in football. *Neurosurgery*, 2004a, *55*, 649-655.

Levy ML, Ozgur BM, Berry C, et al. Birth and evolution of the football helmet. *Neurosurgery*, 2004b, *55*, 656-662.

Lovell MR. *Does brief loss of consciousness define concussion severity in athletes?* Paper presented at the annual American Medical Society for Sports Medicine Conference, Orlando, 2002.

Lovell MR. The relevance of neuropsychologic testing for sports-related head injuries. *Current Sports Medicine Reports*, 2002, *1*, 7-11.

Lovell MR, Barr W. American professional football. In Lovell MR, Echemendia RJ, Barth JT, et al. (Eds.), *Traumatic brain injury in sports: An international neuropsychological perspective*. Lisse, The Netherlands: Swets & Zeitlinger, 2004.

Lovell MR, Collins MW. Neuropsychological assessment of the college football player. *Journal of Head Trauma Rehabilitation,* 1998, *13,* 9-26.

Lovell MR, Collins MW, Hawn KL, et al. Does brief loss of consciousness define concussion severity in athletes? *Journal of Athletic Training,* 2002, *37,* Supplement, p. S-11.

Lovell MR, Collins MW, Iverson GL, et al. Recovery from mild concussion in high school athletes. *Journal of Neurosurgery,* 2003, *98,* 295-301.

Lovell MR, Echemendia RJ, Barth JT, Collins, MW. (Eds.). *Traumatic brain injury in sports: An international neuropsychological perspective.* Lisse, The Netherlands: Swets & Zeitlinger, 2004.

Lovell MR, Echemendia RJ, Burke CJ. Professional ice hockey. In Lovell MR, Echemendia RJ, Barth JT, et al. (Eds.), *Traumatic brain injury in sports: An international neuropsychological perspective.* Lisse, The Netherlands: Swets & Zeitlinger, 2004.

Lovell MR, Iverson GL, Collins MW, et al. Does loss of consciousness predict neuropsychological decrements after concussion? *Clinical Journal of Sport Medicine,* 1999, *9,* 193-198.

Macciocchi SN, Barth JT, Alves W, et al. Neuropsychological functioning and recovery after mild head injury in collegiate athletes. *Neurosurgery,* 1996, *39,* 510-514.

Macciocchi SN, Barth JT, Littlefield L, et al. Multiple concussions and neuropsychological functioning in collegiate football players. *Journal of Athletic Training,* 2001, *36,* 303-306.

Maddocks DL, Dicker GD, Saling MM. The assessment of orientation following concussion in athletes. *Clinical Journal of Sport Medicine,* 1995, *5,* 32-35.

Maroon JC, Lovell MR, Norwig J, et al. Cerebral concussion in athletes: Evaluation and neuropsychological testing. *Neurosurgery,* 2000, *47,* 659-669.

Mathews WB. Footballer's migraine. *British Medical Journal,* 1972, *809,* 326-327.

Matser JT, Kessels AG, Jordan BD, et al. Chronic traumatic brain injury in professional soccer players. *Neurology,* 1998, *51,* 791-796.

Matser EJT, Kessels AGH, Lezak MD, et al. Neuropsychological impairment in amateur soccer players. *Journal of the American Medical Association,* 1999, *282,* 971-973.

Matser EJT, Kessels AGH, Lezak MD et al. Acute traumatic brain injury in amateur boxing. *The Physician and Sportsmedicine,* 2000, *28,* 87-92.

Matser JT, Kessels AGH, Lezak MD, et al. A dose-response relation of headers and concussions with cognitive impairment in professional soccer players. *Journal of Clinical and Experimental Neuropsychology,* 2001, *23,* 770-774.

McCrea M. Standardized mental status assessment of sports concussion. *Clinical Journal of Sport Medicine,* 2001, *11,* 176-181.

McCrea M. Standardized mental status testing on the sideline after sport-related concussion. *Journal of Athletic Training,* 2001, *36,* 274-279.

McCrea M, Guskiewicz KM, Marshall SW, et al. Acute effects and recovery time following concussion in collegiate football players: The NCAA concussion study. *Journal of the American Medical Association,* 2003, *290,* 2556-2563.

McCrea M, Hammeke T, Olsen G, et al. Unreported concussion in high school football players: Implications for prevention. *Clinical Journal of Sport Medicine*, 2004, *14*, 13-17.

McCrea M, Kelly JP, Kluge J, et al. Standardized assessment of concussion in football players. *Neurology*, 1997, *48*, 586-588.

McCrea M, Kelly JP, Randolph C, et al. Standardized assessment of concussion (SAC): On-site mental status evaluation of the athlete. *Journal of Head Trauma Rehabilitation*, 1998, *13*, 27-35.

McCrea M, Kelly JP, Randolph C, et al. Immediate neurocognitive effects of concussion. *Neurosurgery*, 2002, *50*, 1032-1040.

McCrory P. The eighth wonder of the world: The mythology of concussion management. *British Journal of Sports Medicine*, 1999, *33*, 136-137.

McCrory P. Do mouthguards prevent concussion? *British Journal of Sports Medicine*, 2001a, *35*, 81-82.

McCrory P. Does second impact syndrome exist? *Clinical Journal of Sport Medicine*, 2001b, *11*, 144-149.

McCrory P. New treatments for concussion: The next millennium beckons. *Clinical Journal of Sport Medicine*, 2001c, *11*, 190-193.

McCrory P. When to retire after concussion? *British Journal of Sports Medicine*, 2001d, *35*, 380-382.

McCrory P. Treatment of recurrent concussion. *Current Sports Medicine Reports*, 2002, *1*, 28-32.

McCrory P. Preparticipation assessment for head injury. *Clinical Journal of Sport Medicine*, 2004, *14*, 139-144.

McCrory PR, Berkovic SF. Concussion: The history of clinical and pathophysiological concepts and misconceptions. *Neurology*, 2001, *57*, 2283-2288.

McCrory PR, Berkovic SF, Cordner SM. Deaths due to brain injury among footballers in Victoria, 1968-1999. *Medical Journal of Australia*, 2000, *172*, 217-219.

McCrory P, Collie A, Anderson V, et al. Can we manage sport-related concussion in children the same as in adults? *British Journal of Sports Medicine*, 2004, *38*, 516-519.

McCrory PR, Johnston KM. Acute clinical symptoms of concussion: Assessing prognostic significance. *The Physician and Sportsmedicine*, 2002, *30*, 43-47.

McCrory P, Johnston KM, Mohtadi NG, et al. Evidence-based review of sport-related concussion: Basic science. *Clinical Journal of Sport Medicine*, 2001, *11*, 160-165.

Moriarity J, Collie A, Olson D, et al. A prospective controlled study of cognitive function during an amateur boxing tournament. *Neurology*, 2004, *62*, 1497-1502.

Moser RS, Schatz P. Enduring effects of concussion in youth athletes. *Archives of Clinical Neuropsychology*, 2002, *17*, 91-100.

Mueller FO. Catastrophic head injuries in high school and collegiate sports. *Journal of Athletic Training*, 2001, *36*, 312-315.

National Collegiate Athletic Association (NCAA). Guideline 2o: Concussion and Second-Impact Syndrome. National Collegiate Athletic Association, June 1994 (revised June 2002). Available at www.ncaa.org.

Naunheim RS, Bayly PV, Standeven J, et al. Linear and angular head accelerations during heading of a soccer ball. *Medicine & Science in Sports & Exercise*, 2003, *35*, 1-7.

Naunheim RS, Standeven J, Richter C, et al. Comparison of impact data in hockey, football, and soccer. *Journal of Trauma*, 2000, *48*, 938-941.

Newman JA. Biomechanics of brain injury in athletes. In Lovell MR, Echemendia RJ, Barth JT, et al. (Eds.), *Traumatic brain injury in sports: An international neuropsychological perspective*. Lisse, The Netherlands: Swets & Zeitlinger, 2004.

Olvey SE, Knox T, Cohn KA. The development of a method to measure head acceleration and motion in high-impact crashes. *Neurosurgery*, 2004, *54*, 672-677.

Pashby T, Carson JD, Ordogh D, et al. Eliminate head-checking in ice hockey. *Clinical Journal of Sport Medicine*, 2001, *11*, 211-213.

Pellman EJ, Viano DC, Tucker AM, et al. Concussion in professional football: Reconstruction of game impacts and injuries—Part 1. *Neurosurgery*, 2003a, *53*, 799-812.

Pellman EJ, Viano DC, Tucker AM, et al. Concussion in professional football: Location and direction of helmet impacts—Part 2. *Neurosurgery*, 2003b, *53*, 1328-1340.

Pellman EJ, Powell JW, Viano DC, et al. Concussion in professional football: Epidemiological features of game injuries and review of the literature—Part 3. *Neurosurgery*, 2004a, *54*, 81-94.

Pellman EJ, Viano DC, Casson IR, et al. Concussion in professional football: Repeat injuries—Part 4. *Neurosurgery*, 2004b, *55*, 860-876.

Pellman EJ, Viano DC, Casson IR, et al. Concussion in professional football: Injuries involving 7 or more days out—Part 5. *Neurosurgery*, 2004c, *55*, 1100-1119.

Pellman EJ, Viano DC, Casson IR, et al. Concussion in professional football: Players returning to same game—Part 7. *Neurosurgery*, 2005, *56*, 79-90.

Peterson CL, Ferrara MS, Mrazik M, et al. Evaluation of neuropsychological domain scores and postural stability following cerebral concussion in sports. *Clinical Journal of Sport Medicine*, 2003, *13*, 230-237.

Piland SG, Motl RW, Ferrara MS, et al. Evidence for the factorial and construct validity of a self-report concussion symptoms scale. *Journal of Athletic Training*, 2003, *38*, 104-112.

Plassman BL, Havilk RJ, Steffens DC, et al. Documented head injury in early adulthood and risk of Alzheimer's disease and other dementias. *Neurology*, 2000, *55*, 1158-1166.

Podell K. *Computerized assessment of sports-related brain injury*. In Lovell MR, Echemendia RJ, Barth JT, et al. (Eds.), *Traumatic brain injury in sports: An international neuropsychological perspective*. Lisse, The Netherlands: Swets & Zeitlinger, 2004.

Porter MD. A 9-year controlled prospective neuropsychologic assessment of amateur boxing. *Clinical Journal of Sport Medicine*, 2003, *13*, 339-352.

Powell JW. Cerebral concussion: Causes, effects, and risks in sports. *Journal of Athletic Training*, 2001, *36*, 307-311.

Powell JW, Barber-Foss KD. Traumatic brain injury in high school athletes. *Journal of the American Medical Association*, 1999, *282*, 958-963.

Powell JW, Dompier TP. The role of the helmet in the prevention of traumatic brain injuries. *Current Sports Medicine Reports*, 2004, *3*, 20-24.

Putukian M. Heading in soccer: Is it safe? *Current Sports Medicine Reports*, 2004, *3*, 9-14.

Putukian M, Echemendia RJ, Evans TA, et al. *Effects of heading contacts in collegiate soccer players on cognitive function: Prospective neuropsychological assessment over a season.* Paper presented at the 10th Annual Meeting of the American Medical Society for Sports Medicine, April, 2001.

Putukian M, Echemendia RJ, Mackin S. The acute neuropsychological effects of heading in soccer: A pilot study. *Clinical Journal of Sport Medicine*, 2000, *10*, 104-109.

Rabadi MH, Jordan BD. The cumulative effect of repetitive concussion in sports. *Clinical Journal of Sport Medicine*, 2001, *11*, 194-198.

Radelet MA, Lephart SM, Rubinstein EN, et al. Survey of the injury rate for children in community sports. *Pediatrics*, 2002, *110*, e28.

Randolph C, Barr WB, McCrea, M. Is neuropsychological testing useful in the management of sport-related concussion? *Journal of Athletic Training*, in press.

Rasmussen AM, Kaminski TW, Horodyski MB, et al. The effects of purposeful heading on postural stability and cognitive functioning in female soccer players. *Journal of Athletic Training*, 2002, *37*, S-S.

Ravdin LD, Barr WB, Jordan B, et al. Assessment of cognitive recovery following sports-related head trauma in boxers. *Clinical Journal of Sport Medicine*, 2003, *13*, 21-27.

Report of the Sports Medicine Committee. Guidelines for the management of concussion in sports. Colorado Medical Society, 1990. (Revised May 1991).

Roberts AH. *Brain damage in boxers*. London: Pitman Medical Scientific, 1969.

Ross S, Guskiewicz KM, Onate J. Symptomatology following cerebral concussion and its relationship with neuropsychological and postural stability tests (Abstract). *Journal of Athletic Training*, 2000, *35*, S53.

Saunders RL, Harbaugh RE. The second impact in catastrophic contact-sports head trauma. *Journal of the American Medical Association*, 1984, *252*, 538-539.

Schneider RC. *Head and neck injuries in football: Mechanisms, treatment, and prevention.* Baltimore: Williams & Wilkins, 1973.

Sortland O, Tysvaer AT. Brain damage in former association football players: An evaluation by cerebral computed tomography. *Neuroradiology*, 1989, *31*, 44-48.

Stalnacke B-M, Tegner Y, Sojka P. Playing ice hockey and basketball increases serum levels of S-100B in elite players: A pilot study. *Clinical Journal of Sport Medicine*, 2003, *13*, 292-302.

Stalnacke B-M, Tegner Y, Sojka P. Playing soccer increases serum concentrations of the biochemical markers of brain damage S-100B and neuron-specific enolase in elite players: A pilot study. *Brain Injury*, 2004, *18*, 899-909.

Steffens DC, Skoog I, Norton MC, et al. Prevalence of depression and its treatment in an elderly population: The Cache County study. *Archives of General Psychiatry*, 2000, *57*, 601-607.

Sundstrom A, Marklund P, Nilsson LG, et al. ApoE influences on neuropsychological function after mild head injury. *Neurology,* 2004, *62,* 1963-1966.

Tagliabue P. Tackling concussions in sports. *Neurosurgery,* 2003, *53,* 796.

Teasdale G, Jennett B. Assessment of coma and impaired consciousness: A practical scale. *Lancet,* 1974, *2,* 81-84.

Tegeler, C. *New developments in clinical neuroscience.* Paper presented at the New Developments in Sports-Related Concussion Conference, Pittsburgh, July 2004.

Thorndike A. Serious recurrent injuries of athletes. *New England Journal of Medicine,* 1952, *246,* 554-556.

Torg JS, Vegso JJ, Sennett B, et al. The national football head and neck injury registry: 14-year report on cervical quadriplegia, 1971 through 1984. *Journal of the American Medical Association,* 1985, *254,* 3439-3443.

Tysvaer AT. Head and neck injuries in soccer: Impact of minor trauma. *Sports Medicine,* 1992, *14,* 200-213.

Tysvaer AT, Storli OV. Soccer injuries to the brain: A neurologic and electroencephalographic study of active football players. *American Journal of Sports Medicine,* 1989, *17,* 573-578.

Tysvaer AT, Storli OV, Bachen NI. Soccer injuries to the brain: A neurologic and electroencephalographic study of former players. *Acta Neurologica Scandinavia,* 1989, *80,* 151-156.

Tysvaer AT, Lochen EA. Soccer injuries to the brain. *American Journal of Sports Medicine,* 1991, *19,* 56-60.

Valovich TC, Perrin DH, Gansneder BM. Repeat administration elicits a practice effect with the Balance Error Scoring System but not with the Standardized Assessment of Concussion in high school athletes. *Journal of Athletic Training,* 2003, *38,* 51-56.

Vos PE, Lamers KJ, Hendriks JC, et al. Glial and neuronal proteins in serum predict outcome after severe traumatic brain injury. *Neurology,* 2004, *62,* 1303-1310.

Wennberg RA, Tator CH. National Hockey League reported concussions, 1986-87 to 2001-02. *Canadian Journal of Neurological Sciences,* 2003, *30,* 206-209.

Wilkins JC, McLeod TC, Perrin DH, et al. Performance on the Balance Error Scoring System decreases after fatigue. *Journal of Athletic Training,* 2004, *39,* 156-161.

Winters JE. Commentary: Role of properly fitted mouthguards in prevention of sport-related concussion. *Journal of Athletic Training,* 2001, *36,* 339-341.

Witol AD, Webbe, FM. Soccer heading frequency predicts neuropsychological deficits. *Archives of Clinical Neuropsychology,* 2003, *18,* 397-417.

Wojtys EM, Hovda D, Landry G, et al. Concussion in sports. *American Journal of Sports Medicine,* 1999, *27,* 676-687.

Yarnell PR, Lynch S. The "ding": Amnestic states in football trauma. *Neurology,* 1973, *23,* 196-197.

Zariczny B, Shattuck LJ, Mast TA, et al. Sports-related injuries in school-age children. *American Journal of Sports Medicine,* 1980, *8,* 318-324.

About the Authors

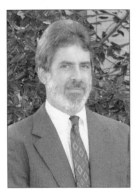

Gary S. Solomon, PhD, is a member of Psychiatric Consultants, P.C., a behavioral health group in Nashville. He is the team neuropsychologist for the National Hockey League Nashville Predators and a consulting neuropsychologist for the National Football League Tennessee Titans. A member of the American Neuropsychiatric Association and the International Neuropsychological Society, he did his dissertation on head injuries and has treated patients with head injuries for more than 20 years. Certified by the American Board of Professional Neuropsychology, he is a fellow of the National Academy of Neuropsychology.

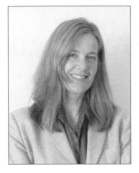

Karen M. Johnston, MD, PhD, is the director of the Concussion Program at McGill Sport Medicine Centre and a Neurosurgeon with the McGill University Health Centre in Montreal, Quebec. She is the Chair of the Concussion in Sport Group, International Olympic Committee, Fédération Internationale de Football Association, and the International Ice Hockey Federation, in addition to serving as the Neurosurgeon/Consultant for organizations such as the National Hockey League Players Association, the Canadian Football League, and others. She is chair of the Concussion Education Program and vice president of Think First.

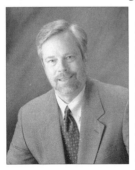

Mark R. Lovell, PhD, is an assistant professor of orthopaedics at the University of Pittsburgh and director of the University of Pittsburgh Sports Medicine Concussion Program. He serves as the neuropsychological consultant for organizations such as the Pittsburgh Steelers Football Club, the Pittsburgh Penguins Hockey Club, the International Olympic Committee, and the International Ice Hockey Federation. Lovell is a reviewer of *The Journal of Neuropsychiatry and Clinical Neuroscience* and *The Journal of Athletic Training*.